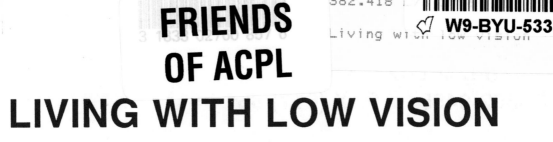
LIVING WITH LOW VISION

A Resource Guide

for

People with Sight Loss

Resources for Rehabilitation
Lexington, Massachusetts

Resources for Rehabilitation
33 Bedford Street, Suite 19A
Lexington, MA 02173
(617) 862-6455   FAX (617) 861-7517

ISBN 0-929718-14-3

For a complete list of publications by Resources for Rehabilitation, see pages 285-288 of this book.

TABLE OF CONTENTS

INTRODUCTION

This book was written to inform people with vision loss about the many organizations and assistive devices that can help them to remain independent. The services and products that enable people with vision loss to keep working, reading, and carrying out their daily activities have proliferated in recent years. Unfortunately, many people with vision loss never learn about these services or products and therefore are unable to achieve their maximum level of independence. Since people have different lifestyles and different degrees of sight loss, inevitably they will need different services to remain independent. This book is organized to enable individuals to select the services and products that are most appropriate to their specific needs.

Each chapter includes an introductory narrative, information about national organizations that provide services to individuals with vision loss and to members of their families, and information about relevant publications. Only directories that have timely information and those that are updated regularly are included. Unless otherwise noted, all publications are in standard print and all videotapes are produced in VHS format.

Descriptions of organizations, publications and tapes, and assistive devices are alphabetical within sections. Although many of the publications described are available in libraries or bookstores, the addresses and phone numbers of publishers and distributors are included for those who wish to purchase the books by mail or phone. All of the material is up-to-date, and prices were accurate at the time of publication. All prices are quoted in U.S. dollars unless otherwise noted. It is always advisable to contact publishers and manufacturers to inquire about availability and current prices.

Developments in computer technology such as bulletin boards, e-mail, and the Internet have greatly increased access to information for the general population as well as people with low vision. E-mail and Internet addresses are given for many organizations listed in this book. Since changes and additions are frequent, readers should check bulletin boards regularly for updates.

KEY TO ABBREVIATIONS AND TERMINOLOGY

B = braille

BBS = bulletin board service accessible with PC, modem, telephone, and communication software

C = audiocassette

4-track audiocassette = must be played on NLS or alternate brand 4-track cassette players

disc = must be played on NLS slow speed record player

LP = large print

P = standard print*

PC = personal computer (IBM or compatible)

TT = text telephone, special telephone system for individuals who are deaf or have hearing impairments and those who have speech impairments (formerly known as TDD, telecommunication device for the deaf)

V = telephone number for voice communication

V/TT = same telephone number for voice or text telephone

* Unless otherwise noted, all publications listed are available in standard print. This abbreviation is used only when a publication is available in standard print as well as other formats.

The following are terms used to access Internet resources:
e-mail
gopher
http://
telnet
www (world wide web)

Chapter 1

EXPERIENCING VISION LOSS

The number of individuals experiencing vision loss in industrialized countries is increasing, due in large part to the aging of the population. According to the U.S. Bureau of the Census, nearly 10 million Americans age 15 or older have reported that they have difficulty reading words and letters in ordinary newsprint even when wearing corrective lenses; 1.6 million could not see words or letters at all (McNeil: 1993). In Canada, over one-half million individuals age 15 or older are unable to read ordinary newsprint or to see someone from four meters (Statistics Canada: 1988). In both countries, visual impairment is most prevalent among those age 65 years or older.

The experience of vision loss brings with it a variety of emotions, ranging from fear and denial to acceptance and adjustment. Such emotions are normal. An individual's response to vision loss will be based on coping mechanisms that have been developed over the course of a lifetime. Obtaining adequate information about the condition that caused the vision loss and the prognosis; locating professional service providers that elicit confidence; and talking to peers who have experienced vision loss may play a significant role in adjusting to vision loss and functioning independently.

This chapter provides basic information about vision loss, terminology, and resources that can help people

LIVING WITH LOW VISION: A Resource Guide for People with Sight Loss, Lexington, MA: Resources for Rehabilitation, Copyright 1996

cope with everyday activities and emotional responses to vision loss.

DEFINITIONS OF VISION LOSS

Two types of visual impairment are central vision loss and peripheral or field loss. Central vision loss causes difficulties with tasks that require fine, detailed vision, such as reading and recognizing faces. Peripheral vision loss, sometimes called tunnel vision, causes problems with mobility. Since the visual field is restricted, a person with this type of vision loss may be able to see only part of a page, face, or scene.

Low vision is the term that is commonly used to refer to visual impairments that leave the individual with some residual vision. Although there are no standard definitions of low vision, professionals usually consider an acuity of 20/70 or worse in the better eye to be low vision. Low vision may be moderate or severe.

In the U.S., individuals are considered to be legally blind if they have a visual acuity of 20/200 or worse in the better eye with all possible correction (glasses) or a visual field of 20 degrees diameter or less (tunnel vision) in the better eye. Most individuals who are legally blind retain some useful vision and should be encouraged to use it to the maximum extent possible. The classification of legal blindness entitles U.S. citizens to tax benefits and to rehabilitation services provided by state governments. Definitions of legal blindness vary in other countries.

OBTAINING INFORMATION ABOUT YOUR CONDITION

If you (or your child or other close relative) have experienced irreversible vision loss, you should ask the ophthalmologist about the nature of the disease, the prognosis, and the functional implications of the condition. You should explain what aspects of life have become difficult and ask the ophthalmologist for an appropriate referral.

Failure to ask questions at an initial appointment with the ophthalmologist should not deter you from getting the information you need. Phone the office and schedule a follow-up appointment. Be prepared with a list of questions that you would like to have answered. Write out the questions with a bold point pen or bring along a family member or close friend to make sure that you don't forget anything that you want to ask.

Below are some questions that are meant to serve as guidelines in your discussions with ophthalmologists or other service providers. Not everyone needs or wants the same amount or type of information. The questions below are meant as suggestions only, and each individual must decide what information is useful.

● What is the medical name of the disease or condition that has caused my vision loss? What causes this condition? Do you have any literature or videotapes describing the condition?

● Are any of my other health conditions related to my vision problems? Are the medications I am taking affecting my vision?

- What treatment is currently available? Will this treatment affect my other health conditions?
- If treatment is available, where can I obtain a second opinion (sometimes required for payment by insurance companies)?
- Is there anything I can do that will help prevent further loss of vision?
- What is my acuity? What is my field of vision? Am I legally blind? If so, have you registered me with the state agency that serves people who are visually impaired or blind? (In some states and in Canada, legal blindness is not a prerequisite for receiving services.)
- Is there any activity I should avoid?
- Is it possible that the drugs I am taking for another condition are contributing to my vision problem?
- What groups or organizations exist to serve people with my condition?
- How can I best use my remaining vision? What types of equipment can help me function better?

A vast amount of information is available from medical databases and libraries. MEDLINE, a computerized database of articles in all major medical journals, is operated by the National Library of Medicine (see listing under ORGANIZATIONS section below). It is available through commercial online services as well as through the Internet. Many public libraries now offer MEDLINE access, as do most university and hospital libraries.

It is possible to conduct a MEDLINE search by topic, such as macular degeneration, glaucoma, etc. Although consumers with medical problems may not understand every aspect of the articles they read in medical journals, they may learn enough to pose additional important questions to health care providers and to learn about new experimental treatments and clinical trials sponsored by the National Eye Institute.

In addition, the Internet, often referred to as the information superhighway, provides numerous newsgroups, where consumers may discuss their common problems and solutions, and databases that provide information on new treatments. The reference section of most libraries contains indexes and directories of resources available on the Internet. Look up topics such as disabilities, health, and blindness. Since new resources become available all the time, sometimes it is necessary to browse various services to obtain up-to-date information. A gopher site on the Internet, info.umd.edu, lists disability related Internet resources; choose "academic resources," then "disability resources."

REHABILITATION SERVICES

Rehabilitation services are designed to help people with progressive and/or irreversible impairments continue functioning in society. Rehabilitation services may include any or all of the following:

- rehabilitation counseling
- job placement

- adaptive equipment, prostheses, and medical supplies
- adapting the home or work environment
- vocational training to retain a current position or to learn a new skill
- training in activities of daily living and home-making
- volunteer services
- transportation services

Rehabilitation services are provided by both public and private agencies. In the U.S., each state has a public agency that is responsible for providing vocational rehabilitation services to individuals who are visually impaired or blind. Most states also have private organizations which provide services to individuals with vision loss. Some of these agencies may require that individuals be legally blind in order to receive services, while others serve people with any degree of visual impairment. Some rehabilitation professionals provide services independently on a fee for service basis. Rehabilitation services are offered in group settings, in residential settings, or at home.

Some states require that ophthalmologists and optometrists register individuals who are legally blind with the state agency. Ask your ophthalmologist or optometrist if you are legally blind; if you are, request a letter stating that you are legally blind and ask to be registered with the state agency.

Individuals who are legally blind are eligible for a variety of services as well as certain types of financial benefits. The state agency for individuals who are visually impaired or blind is an important resource, since it often funds medical treatment, specialized equipment, education, training programs, and homemaker services. Ask for a complete description of the agency's services as well as services provided by other public and private organizations.

In addition to vocational rehabilitation services that enable people with vision loss to return to work, many states offer special programs for children and elders. Rehabilitation guidelines have been expanded to include the role of "homemaker" as a justifiable rehabilitation goal. The services for elders with visual impairment are often called Independent Living Programs (ILP). These programs have the goal of enabling individuals to remain independent, whether or not they expect to continue working. ILP's vary in their settings, structures, and the types of services they offer. They may be operated by rehabilitation agencies or as independent entities.

For individuals who are not legally blind, there are alternative options available. If the state agency serves only individuals who are legally blind, ask the public information officer for suggestions about other organizations that serve individuals who have lost vision but are not legally blind. In some states, departments serving elders arrange for services to individuals who are not legally blind (See Chapter 8, "SERVICES FOR ELDERS"). Many ophthalmologists' and optometrists' offices offer low vision services, as do some residential schools for blind children (See Chapter 9, "SERVICES FOR CHILDREN AND ADOLESCENTS").

A wide variety of services is offered to Canadians

with any degree of vision loss through the offices of the Canadian National Institute for the Blind (CNIB), a private, nonprofit organization. CNIB offers services for Canadians of all ages, a national library service, and special services for people who are deaf-blind, veterans, and individuals with multiple disabilities. (See the listing for the main office of CNIB below and Appendix B: Division Offices of the Canadian National Institute for the Blind.) Most provinces also have other private organizations which provide services to individuals with vision loss.

LOW VISION SERVICES

Low vision services, sometimes called low vision clinics, are operated by ophthalmologists, optometrists, or other professionals who have been specially trained in low vision. Professionals in low vision services assess their clients' visual functioning and how it affects their daily activities. Individuals who wear eyeglasses or contact lenses should have an accurate and up-to-date refraction prior to receiving low vision aids.

Aids and devices that can improve functioning for specific activities are prescribed for the client. Some low vision services prescribe only optical or nonoptical aids, while others are multidisciplinary and include orientation and mobility training, rehabilitation teaching, and in-dividual, family, and/or peer counseling.

Many low vision services require a referral from an ophthalmologist or optometrist along with results of a recent ophthalmological exam. Before making an appointment at a low vision service, be certain to ask about the types of services provided. Some low vision services allow clients to borrow aids for a specified period of time prior to purchase. Especially in the case of expensive aids, it is wise to ask for such a trial period.

Low vision services are often available in public or private agencies serving individuals who are visually impaired or blind, in ophthalmology departments at hospitals, private ophthalmologists' or optometrists' offices, colleges of optometry, or schools for the blind. In some cases, low vision services are independent organizations.

In many instances, health insurance does not cover the cost of aids prescribed at low vision services. Check with your insurance company prior to purchase. Also check with the public agency in your area to determine if it will provide low vision aids or reimburse you for aids purchased privately. Most vocational rehabilitation agencies must provide their approval before a low vision evaluation is performed if they are to reimburse the low vision specialists. Some community service organizations such as Lions Clubs, Knights Templar, etc. will purchase aids for local residents. The staff at the low vision service should be able to provide information about these organizations.

PROFESSIONAL SERVICE PROVIDERS

There are many professionals who provide crucial services to people with vision loss. It is important for all professionals to be aware of the services provided by other professionals, in order to coordinate a plan of health care and rehabilitation.

An OPHTHALMOLOGIST (M.D.) is a physician who specializes in diseases of the eye and systemic diseases that affect the eye's functioning. Ophthalmologists should refer patients for rehabilitation services when medical or surgical treatment cannot restore vision to normal levels. An OPTOMETRIST (O.D.) is trained to conduct refractions and prescribe corrective lenses. In some states, optometrists are also licensed to prescribe drugs. An OPTICIAN is trained to make and dispense corrective lenses. A LOW VISION SPECIALIST may be an ophthalmologist, optometrist, optician, or other professional who is trained to help individuals with vision loss use their remaining vision to the greatest extent possible with the assistance of optical and nonoptical aids.

A REHABILITATION COUNSELOR serves as a case coordinator for individuals who are visually impaired or blind and require rehabilitation services. The rehabilitation counselor helps the individual to establish a work plan (Individual Written Rehabilitation Plan or IWRP) that is appropriate, realistic, and agreed upon by the counselor and the individual. (See Chapter 5, "HOW TO KEEP WORKING WITH VISION LOSS.")

A REHABILITATION TEACHER conducts a functional assessment and provides individualized instruction in activities of daily living. This instruction may include practical adaptations such as LARGE PRINT telephone numbers; markers for stoves, thermostats, and medications; and suggestions to increase home safety. The rehabilitation teacher also provides information about community resources and services.

An ORIENTATION AND MOBILITY (O and M) instructor orients the individual to his or her home and teaches safe travel skills in the immediate areas outside the home and along commonly traveled routes, to the workplace, supermarket, or senior center.

A SPECIAL EDUCATOR or VISION TEACHER works with parents to develop special education services for children who are visually impaired or blind. (See Chapter 9, "SERVICES FOR CHILDREN AND ADOLESCENTS," for a more detailed explanation of the role of these professionals.)

An OCCUPATIONAL THERAPIST (OT) is trained to assess the home, school, and work environment and to suggest environmental adaptations and adaptive aids. The goal of occupational therapists is to teach individuals with vision loss and other disabilities how to become independent in their everyday activities. Occupational therapists may work in hospitals, rehabilitation agencies, schools, industry, or in private practices.

Other health professionals who may be involved in providing services are internists or general practitioners, diabetologists, physical therapists, audiologists, and mental health professionals such as psychologists, psychiatrists, social workers, and other counselors.

COMPUTERS AND LOW VISION

Personal computers (PCs) have opened up a wide variety of opportunities for people who are visually impaired or blind. Used alone, adapted PCs enable individuals to obtain files that may be output in LARGE

PRINT, speech, or braille. Throughout this book are references to bulletin board services operated by agencies as well as Internet resources. Using PCs with the Internet, online subscription services, or bulletin board services (usually run by a community service agency), individuals are able to communicate with people all over the world. This instant communication provides up-to-the-minute information about new developments and the opportunity to "chat" with individuals in similar situations. Many of these services are free, with the exception of telephone charges or subscription fees for online services.

HOW TO FIND SERVICES

The telephone directory or information operator can help you find the services available in your area. Some telephone directories have a section called "Community Services Numbers: A Self-Help Guide," which lists many agencies and their toll-free numbers. If there are government listings in the local phone book, look for the Citizens Information Service for federal, state, and city agencies. Services for people with low vision may be provided by a "Commission for the Blind," "State Services for the Blind," "Department of Rehabilitation," or may be listed under a Department of Education or Labor. The state government information operator can help you locate the appropriate agency in your state. Don't be put off if agencies have the word "blind" in their names; they often deal with many forms of vision problems, from low vision to eye diseases which are controlled with medication.

Other good places to learn about services are the

public library (ask the reference librarian for local service directories); a local or state medical, ophthalmology, or optometry society; the social services department or the patient education department of a hospital; and the local United Way office.

This Resource Guide will help you to discover the wide variety of services, self-help groups, products, and publications that can enable you to make the best use of your remaining vision.

REFERENCES

McNeil, John M.
1993 AMERICANS WITH DISABILITIES 1991-1992, Washington, DC: U.S. Bureau of the Census Current Population Reports P70-33

Statistics Canada
1988 THE HEALTH AND ACTIVITY LIMITATION SURVEY: USER'S GUIDE, Ottawa, Canada

NATIONAL SOURCES OF INFORMATION

ORGANIZATIONS

ALLIANCE OF GENETIC SUPPORT GROUPS
35 Wisconsin Circle, Suite 440
Chevy Chase, MD 20815
(800) 336-4363   (301) 652-5553
FAX (301) 654-0171

Provides education and services to families and individuals affected by genetic disorders. Monthly news bulletin, "Alert." Membership, individuals, $20.00; organizations, $50.00.

AMERICAN COUNCIL OF THE BLIND (ACB)
1155 15th Street NW, Suite 720
Washington, DC 20005
(800) 424-8666   (202) 467-5081
FAX (202) 467-5085   BBS (202) 331-1058

Membership organization with chapters in many states. Special interest groups such as blind parents, guide dog users, low vision, students, etc. The "Washington Connection," a recorded message about legislation, is available daily, from 6 pm to midnight, E.S.T., and weekends by calling the toll-free number. Publishes the "Braille Forum," a monthly newsletter in LP, C, B, and PC disk. Membership, $5.00.

AMERICAN FOUNDATION FOR THE BLIND (AFB)
11 Penn Plaza, Suite 300
New York, NY 10001
(212) 502-7600   FAX (212) 502-7774
Information line (800) 232-5463
In NY, (212) 502-7657

An information clearinghouse on blindness and visual impairment. "Publications Catalog," FREE.

CANADIAN NATIONAL INSTITUTE FOR THE BLIND (CNIB)
National Office
1929 Bayview Avenue
Toronto, Ontario M4G 3E8 Canada
(416) 480-7580   FAX (416) 480-7677

CNIB provides seven core services to Canadians with any degree of functional vision impairment: counseling and referral, rehabilitation teaching, orientation and mobility, sight enhancement, technical aids, career development, and library services. Operates resource centres and technology centres and provides special services for seniors, veterans, and people who are deaf-blind. Public information literature available. See Appendix B: Division Offices of the Canadian National Institute for the Blind for addresses of provincial offices.

COMBINED HEALTH INFORMATION DATABASE (CHID)
Box CHID
Bethesda, MD 20892
(301) 468-2162

A federally sponsored database for service providers and consumers; includes bibliographic citations and abstracts from journals, reports, and education programs. Special files on eye health, diabetes, etc. Available at many libraries or services may be purchased for use on a personal computer.

COUNCIL OF CITIZENS WITH LOW VISION INTERNATIONAL (CCLVI)
5707 Brockton Drive, #302
Indianapolis, IN 46220-5481
(800) 733-2258   (317) 254-1185
FAX (317) 251-6588

Provides support, education, and advocacy. Membership, U.S., $10.00; Canada, $10.00; institutions, $25.00; foreign, $30.00; includes "Vision Access," a quarterly newsletter; LP and C. CCLVI offers three bulletin boards for computer users. Contact office for details.

NATIONAL ASSOCIATION FOR VISUALLY HANDICAPPED (NAVH)
22 West 21st Street
New York, NY 10010
(212) 889-3141

Sells LP books and low vision aids. Produces two LP newsletters, "Seeing Clearly," and "In Focus" (for youth), both FREE. Membership, $40.00, includes discounts on purchases and use of library; limited membership, $25.00 (no library privileges). FREE catalogue.

NATIONAL EYE INSTITUTE (NEI)
Building 31, Room 6A32
Bethesda, MD 20892
(301) 496-5248

Conducts basic and clinical research on the causes and cures of eye diseases. Distributes brochures on eye diseases and conditions, such as age-related macular degeneration, cataract, diabetic retinopathy, and glaucoma; FREE. NEI also recruits patients as subjects for a variety of clinical studies. Referrals from ophthalmologists are necessary for enrollment in an appropriate study.

NATIONAL FEDERATION OF THE BLIND (NFB)
1800 Johnson Street
Baltimore, MD 21230
(410) 659-9314   FAX (410) 685-5653

National membership organization with chapters in many states. Provides information about available services, laws, and evaluation of new technology. Special interest groups for students, parents of blind children, etc. Holds state and national annual conventions. Publishes the "Braille Monitor," a monthly magazine; P, C, disc, and B. $25.00 per year contribution requested.

NATIONAL LIBRARY OF CANADA (NLC)
395 Wellington Street
Ottawa, Ontario K1A 0N4 Canada
(613) 996-7504   FAX (613) 947-2706

National library service that serves Canadian residents through interlibrary loan. Houses a collection of books in LARGE PRINT, braille, and audiocassette. Maintains CAN-UC:H, a catalogue of library materials available in special formats such as braille, LARGE PRINT, e-text, talking books, and open and closed captioned videos.

NATIONAL LIBRARY OF MEDICINE (NLM)
8600 Rockville Pike
Building 38, Room 2S-10
Bethesda, MD 20894
(800) 272-4787   (301) 496-6095

Operates MEDLINE, a computerized database of articles in major medical journals from around the world. Users may search for a specific health related topic and receive citations and abstracts of articles. Available directly through NLM and through the Internet, subscription services, and at most medical, public, and university libraries.

NATIONAL LIBRARY SERVICE FOR THE BLIND AND PHYSICALLY HANDICAPPED (NLS)
1291 Taylor Street, NW
Washington, DC 20542
(800) 424-8567 or 8572 (Reference Section)
(800) 424-9100 (to receive application)
(202) 707-5100 FAX (202) 707-0712
telnet marvel.loc.gov (log in as marvel, select Library of Congress Online Systems, select connect to LOCIS, then select "Braille and Audio" for a catalogue of braille and tape publications)

National library service that serves individuals in the U.S. and U.S. residents living abroad. Regional libraries in many states. Individuals must be unable to read standard print due to visual impairment or physical disability. "Facts: Books for Blind and Physically Handicapped Individuals" describes NLS programs and eligibility requirements. Order form lists general information brochures, magazines and newsletters, directories, reference circulars, and subject and reference bibliographies. "Talking Book Topics," published bimonthly, in LP, C, and disc, lists titles recently added to the national collection which are available through the network of regional libraries. All services and publications from NLS are FREE (See Chapter 4, "READING WITH VISION LOSS.")

NATIONAL ORGANIZATION FOR RARE DISORDERS (NORD)
100 Rt. 37, PO Box 8923
New Fairfield, CT 06812-1783
(203) 746-6518   CompuServe "GO NORD"

Federation of voluntary health organizations that serve individuals with rare or "orphan" diseases, including diseases and conditions that affect vision. Reprints of articles on rare diseases available from the NORD Rare Disease Database for $4.00 per copy. Publishes newsletter, "Orphan Disease Update," three times per year, FREE. Membership, $25.00.

NATIONAL REHABILITATION INFORMATION CENTER (NARIC)
8455 Colesville Road, Suite 935
Silver Spring, MD 20910-3319
(800) 346-2742 (V/TT)   (301) 588-9284 (V/TT)
FAX (301) 587-1967   BBS (301) 589-3563
telnet fedworld.gov (select 8, then 1, then 115)

A federally funded center that responds to inquiries about disabilities and support services. Newsletter, "NARIC Quarterly," FREE.

PREVENT BLINDNESS AMERICA
500 East Remington Road
Schaumburg, IL 60173
(800) 331-2020   (708) 843-2020
FAX (708) 843-8458

Sponsors vision screenings. Local and state affiliates. Publications related to diseases and eye injuries, including some in Spanish. FREE catalogue. Newsletter, "Prevent Blindness News," FREE.

RESOURCES FOR REHABILITATION
33 Bedford Street, Suite 19A
Lexington, MA 02173
(617) 862-6455   FAX (617) 861-7517

Conducts programs to educate the public and professionals about the needs of people with vision loss and the resources available to meet those needs. Write or call to arrange special programs at your institution or to be notified about programs in your area.

Produces the "Living with Low Vision" series, including LARGE PRINT (18 point bold) publications that describe service organizations, publications, and products for people with vision loss. Titles include "Living with Low Vision," "How to Keep Reading with Vision Loss," "Aids for Everyday Living," and a series of disease specific publications. Minimum purchase, 25 copies per title. See pages 285-288 of this book for complete publication list.

UNITED WAY OF AMERICA (UWA)
701 North Fairfax Street
Alexandria, VA 22314-2045
(703) 836-7100

UNITED WAY/CENTRAIDE CANADA
56 Spark Street, Suite 404
Ottawa, Ontario K1P 5A9 Canada
(613) 236-7041   FAX (613) 236-3087

An umbrella organization which links local human service organizations. Look in the phone book for the United Way in your area. National offices in the U.S. and Canada can direct you to the local UW, which in turn will provide referral to specific services in your community.

VISION FOUNDATION, INC.
818 Mt. Auburn Street
Watertown, MA 02172
(617) 926-4232   In MA, (800) 852-3029
FAX (617) 926-1412

Information center for individuals with sight loss. Publishes materials in LP and C, including the VISION Resource List (FREE) and "VISION Resource Update," a bimonthly resource newsletter (membership benefit). Membership, fixed income, $15.00; individuals, $30.00; families, $40.00.

PUBLICATIONS AND TAPES

COPING WITH LOW VISION
by Marshall E. Flax, Don J. Golembiewski and Bette L. McCaulley
Singular Publishing Group, Inc.
4284 41st Street
San Diego, CA 92105-1197
(800) 521-8545   FAX (800) 774-8398

This book discusses low vision, vision rehabilitation services, low vision aids, and community resources. Includes resource list of organizations in the U.S. and Canada. LP, $18.95. Also available on 4-track audiocassette from National Library Service for the Blind and Physically Handicapped regional libraries, RC 38113.

COPING WITH THE DIAGNOSIS OF SIGHT LOSS
Resources for Rehabilitation
33 Bedford Street, Suite 19A
Lexington, MA 02173
(617) 862-6455   FAX (617) 861-7517

Three consumers discuss their reactions and experiences when told that they were losing their vision. C, $12.00 plus $3.00 shipping and handling.

THE ENCOUNTER
Carmichael Audio-Video Duplication
1025 South Saddleback Creek Road
Omaha, NE 68106
(402) 556-5677   FAX (402) 556-5416

A videotape about interactions between people with normal vision and those who are blind, produced by the Nebraska Department of Public Institutions. The tape uses humor to show how people who are blind are capable of independent activities; it also addresses education and employment opportunities. 11 minutes. $8.50

THE FIRST STEPS: HOW TO HELP PEOPLE WHO ARE LOSING THEIR SIGHT
Peninsula Center for the Blind
4151 Middlefield Road
Palo Alto, CA 94303
(415) 858-0202
In CA, from area code 408, (800) 660-2009

A booklet written to answer some of the initial questions and discuss some of the initial reactions people have when blindness first occurs in a family. $12.95

A GUIDE TO INDEPENDENCE FOR THE VISUALLY IMPAIRED AND THEIR FAMILIES
by Vivian Younger and Jill Sardegna
Demos Publications
386 Park Avenue South, Suite 201
New York, NY 10016
(800) 532-8663   (212) 683-0072

Written by a vocational counselor who is visually impaired and a writer on disability issues, this book provides practical information for individuals and their families about living independently with vision loss. P, C, and disk (DOS and Mac); $19.95 plus $4.00 shipping and handling.

HOW DO I DO THIS WHEN I CAN'T SEE WHAT I'M DOING? INFORMATION PROCESSING FOR THE VISUALLY DISABLED
by Gerald Jahoda
Superintendent of Documents
PO Box 371954
Pittsburgh, PA 15250-7954
(202) 512-1800   FAX (202) 512-2250
telnet federal.bbs.gpo.gov (Port 3001)
BBS (202) 512-1387

The author, who is blind due to retinitis pigmentosa, describes his own experiences in developing new ways to conduct everyday activities at home and at work. Available in U.S. Government Bookstores. S/N 030-000-00248-2 $5.50. Also available on 4-track audiocassette from National Library Service for the Blind and Physically

Handicapped regional libraries, RC 36212.

IF BLINDNESS STRIKES: DON'T STRIKE OUT
by Margaret Smith
Charles C. Thomas, Publisher
2600 South First Street
Springfield, IL 62794-9265
(800) 258-8980   (217) 789-8980
FAX (217) 789-9130

Written by a rehabilitation counselor who is visually impaired, this book describes many adaptations and strategies for living with vision loss. Hardcover, $46.95; softcover, $29.95; plus $5.50 shipping and handling. Also available on 4-track audiocassette on loan from the National Library Service for the Blind and Physically Handicapped regional libraries, RC 21060. To purchase two-track ($13.50) or 4-track ($7.50) audiocassettes, contact Readings for the Blind, 29451 Greenfield Road, Suite 216, Southfield, MI 48076; (810) 557-7776.

INDEPENDENT LIVING
Equal Opportunity Publications
150 Motor Parkway, Suite 420
Hauppauge, NY 11788
(516) 273-8743   FAX (516) 273-8936

A magazine that addresses the needs of individuals with disabilities in everyday life, including careers and health care issues. Articles written by professionals and consumers. Published seven times a year, including one

issue that is a "Resource Directory & Buyer's Guide."
$18.00

LIVING WITH VISION LOSS

Canadian National Institute for the Blind (CNIB)
1929 Bayview Avenue
Toronto, Ontario M4G 3E8
(416) 480-7626   FAX (416) 480-7677

A videotape with information on causes of visual impairment and adaptations for everyday life including lighting, kitchen skills, and travel. 13 minutes. VHS, $45.00; BETA, $45.00; Canadian funds.

LIVING WITH VISION LOSS: A HANDBOOK FOR CAREGIVERS

Canadian National Institute for the Blind (CNIB)
Rehabilitation Department
1929 Bayview Avenue
Toronto, Ontario M4G 3E8
(416) 480-7626   FAX (416) 480-7677

Practical suggestions for everyday living with visual impairment or blindness. Includes community and CNIB resources. $12.50, Canadian funds.

MAKING LIFE MORE LIVABLE

by Irving R. Dickman
American Foundation for the Blind (AFB)
c/o American Book Center
Brooklyn Navy Yard, Building No. 3
Brooklyn, NY 11205
(718) 852-9873   FAX (718) 935-9647

Offers simple adaptations to make the home safer for people with vision impairment. $16.95 plus $3.50 shipping and handling. Also available on 4-track audiocassette on loan through regional branches of the National Library Service for the Blind and Physically Handicapped. RC 22319.

MOM CAN'T SEE ME
MOM'S BEST FRIEND

by Sally Hobart Alexander
Simon & Schuster
200 Old Tappan Road
Old Tappan, NJ 07675
(800) 223-2336   FAX (800) 445-6991

Written from her nine year old daughter's point of view, the author describes family life with a mother who is blind in MOM CAN'T SEE ME and in MOM'S BEST FRIEND, how she uses a guide dog. LP. $14.95 each.

US AND THEM
Fanlight Productions
47 Halifax Street
Boston, MA 02130
(800) 937-4113   (617) 524-0980
FAX (617) 524-8838

Videotape about relationships between people who have disabilities and those who do not. Includes segment on the relationship between a blind husband and a sighted wife. 32 minutes, black and white. Regular purchase price, $275.00; rental for one day $50.00; for one week $100.00; plus $9.00 shipping charge; call for possible discount.

Chapter 2

LAWS THAT AFFECT PEOPLE WITH VISION LOSS

(For laws specifically related to children and education, see Chapter 9, "CHILDREN AND ADOLESCENTS.")

Laws affecting people with vision loss and other disabilities cover a wide range of issues, including health care, financial benefits, housing, rehabilitation, civil rights, transportation, access to public buildings, and employment. For those who are not specialists in the law, it is sometimes difficult to keep abreast of the laws and their amendments. At the same time, people with disabilities may be able to continue living independently if they are aware of their rights and know how to locate the proper equipment and professional services. In many instances, government programs provide financial assistance for these needs.

In July, 1990, the Americans with Disabilities Act (ADA) was passed (P.L. 101-336). Considered the most important civil rights legislation in recent years, the ADA defines an individual with a disability as a person who has a physical or mental impairment that substantially limits one or more major activities; someone who has had such an impairment; or someone who is regarded as having such an impairment. The ADA increases the steps employers must take to accommodate employees with disabilities and requires that public accommodations be

LIVING WITH LOW VISION: A Resource Guide for People with Sight Loss, Lexington, MA: Resources for Rehabilitation, Copyright 1996

accessible.

The following are the major provisions of the ADA that affect people who are visually impaired or blind:

- Title I prohibits discrimination against individuals with disabilities who are otherwise qualified for employment and requires that employers make "reasonable accommodations." "Reasonable accommodations" include making existing facilities accessible and job restructuring (e.g., reassignment to a vacant position, modification of equipment, training, provision of interpreters and readers). Employers are protected from "undue hardship" in complying with this provision; the financial situation of the employer and the size and type of business are considered when determining whether an accommodation would constitute "undue hardship." The provisions of this section apply to employers with 15 or more employees.

- Title II prohibits discrimination by public entities (i.e., local and state governments) and requires that individuals with disabilities receive the same rights and benefits of public programs as other individuals. For example, local programs for elders may not discriminate against those elders who have low vision or other disabilities; they are entitled to receive the same benefits of the programs as elder who do not have disabilities.

• Title III requires that public accommodations, businesses, and services be accessible to individuals with disabilities. Public accommodations are broadly defined to include places such as hotels and motels, theatres, museums, schools, shopping centers and stores, banks, restaurants, and professionals' offices. Since January 26, 1993, most new construction for public accommodations must be accessible to individuals with disabilities. For example, "raised and brailled characters and pictorial symbol signs" must meet requirements for size, finish, contrast, and mounting location.

• Requires that bus and railroad transportation systems address the needs of individuals with disabilities by purchasing adapted equipment, modifying facilities, and providing special transportation services that are comparable to regular transportation services.

Copies of the ADA are available from Senators and Representatives. In addition, both public agencies and many private agencies that work with individuals who are visually impaired or blind have copies of the ADA available in special formats such as LARGE PRINT, audiocassette, and braille.

Regulations for enforcing individual sections of the act are available from the federal agencies charged with developing them. Agencies charged with formulating regulations and standards include the Architectural and Transportation Barriers Compliance Board, the Department of Transportation, the Equal Employment Opportunity

Commission, and the Attorney General (See "ORGANI-ZATIONS" section below). The Office of the Americans with Disabilities Act within the Department of Justice is responsible for enforcing the ADA.

Individuals who feel that they have been denied employment on the basis of their disability have legal redress, although it is possible to attempt to resolve the dispute through mediation. Legal remedies available to employees or job candidates who believe that their employment rights under the ADA have been violated are those specified under Title VII of the Civil Rights Act of 1964. Administrative enforcement by the Equal Employment Opportunity Commission is the first level of enforcement. After administrative appeals have been exhausted, the right to sue in the federal courts is permitted. Employers violating the law are subject to fines, injunctions ordering compliance, and payment of both back salary and future salary for individuals who have proved discrimination.

The Rehabilitation Act of 1973 (P.L. 93-112) and its amendments are the centerpieces of federal law related to rehabilitation. States must submit a vocational rehabilitation plan to the Rehabilitation Services Administration indicating how the designated state agency will provide vocational training, counseling, and diagnostic and evaluation services required by the law. The "Client Assistance Program" authorizes states to inform clients and other persons with disabilities about all benefits available under the Act and to assist them in obtaining all remedies due under the law (P.L. 98-221).

Section 503 of the Rehabilitation Act requires any

contractor that receives more than $2,500 in contracts from the federal government to take affirmative action to employ individuals with disabilities. The Office of Federal Contract Compliance Programs within the Department of Labor is responsible for enforcing this provision (See "ORGANIZATIONS" section below).

Section 504 prohibits any program that receives federal financial assistance from discriminating against individuals with disabilities who are otherwise eligible to benefit from their programs. Virtually all educational institutions are affected by this law, including private postsecondary institutions which receive federal financial assistance under a wide variety of programs. Programs must be physically accessible to individuals with disabilities, and construction begun after implementation of the regulations (June 3, 1977) must be designed so that it is in compliance with standard specifications for accessibility. Federal agencies must develop an affirmative action plan for hiring, placing, and promoting individuals with disabilities and for making their facilities accessible. The Civil Rights Division of the Department of Justice is responsible for enforcing this section.

"Comprehensive Services for Independent Living" (P.L. 95-602) expanded rehabilitation services to individuals with severe disabilities, regardless of their vocational potential, making services available to many people who are no longer in the work force. The Act broadly defines services as any "service that will enhance the ability of a handicapped individual to live independently or function within his family and community..." These services may include counseling, job placement, housing, funds to make the home accessible, funds for prosthetic devices, attendant care, and recreational activities. The Office of Civil Rights within the Department of Justice enforces the provisions of the Rehabilitation Act.

Supplementary Security Income (SSI) is a federal minimum income maintenance program for elders and individuals who are blind or disabled and who meet a test of financial need. Individuals need not have worked in order to qualify for SSI benefits.

Monthly Social Security Disability Insurance (SSDI) benefits are available to individuals who are disabled and their dependents. To be eligible, individuals must have paid Social Security taxes for a specified number of quarters (dependent upon the applicant's age); must not be working; and must be declared medically disabled by the state disability determination service or through an appeals process. In determining SSDI eligibility for individuals who are legally blind, the quarters of employment which count need not have been earned in the last ten years of work under Social Security. Social Security personnel are sometimes unfamiliar with this policy, described in section RS00301.150A in the "SSDI Program Operating Manual," available in every Social Security office. The disability must be expected to last at least 12 months or to result in death. Individuals who are legally blind and age 55 to 65 may receive monthly benefits if they are unable to carry out the work (or similar work) that they did before age 55 or becoming blind, whichever is later.

Individuals who apply for disability insurance from the Social Security Administration must undergo an evaluation carried out by a state disability evaluation team, composed of physicians, psychologists, and other health care professionals. Social Security disability benefits are not retroactive, so it is important to apply for them immediately after becoming legally blind.

Individuals who have received SSDI for two consecutive years are eligible for Medicare, a federal health insurance program, which may cover some of the necessary out-patient therapy or supplies discussed in this book. However, Medicare does not cover eyeglasses (except following cataract surgery), low vision aids, or hearing aids.

Medicaid is a joint federal/state health insurance plan for individuals who are considered financially needy (i.e., recipients of financial benefits from governmental assistance programs such as Aid to Families with Dependent Children or Supplemental Security Income). While federal law requires that each state cover hospital services, skilled nursing facility services, physician and home health care services, and diagnostic and screening services, states have great discretion in other areas. Payments for prosthetics and rehabilitation equipment vary by state.

The medical and social service benefits available from organizations receiving federal assistance are guaranteed by federal laws and protected by the Office of Civil Rights, Department of Health and Human Services (HHS). When an individual's rights have been violated, a complaint should be filed with the regional office of HHS (See "ORGANIZATIONS" section below).

The Technology-Related Assistance for Individuals with Disabilities Act Amendments of 1994 (P.L. 103-218) strengthened the original Act, passed in 1988. The Act mandated state-wide programs for technology-related assistance to determine needs and resources; to provide technical assistance and information; and to develop demonstration and innovation projects, training programs, and public awareness programs. The amendments set priorities for consumer responsiveness, advocacy, systems change, and outreach to underrepresented populations such as the poor, individuals in rural areas, and minorities.

Under amendments to the Housing and Community Development Act of 1987 (P.L. 100-242), the Department of Housing and Urban Development provides direct loans for the development of projects for elders and individuals with disabilities. These developments may consist of apartments or group homes for up to 15 residents. The Fair Housing Amendments Act of 1988 (P.L. 100-430) requires that multifamily dwellings designed for first occupancy after March 13, 1991 be accessible to individuals with disabilities. In addition, HUD has established programs to house individuals with disabilities who are homeless.

The federal government allows an extra personal exemption on federal income tax for individuals who are legally blind and do not itemize deductions; an extra standard deduction is allowed for those individuals who itemize deductions. Legal blindness is defined as acuity of 20/200 or less in the better eye with the best possible correction or a field of 20 degrees diameter or less in the better eye. Individuals who itemize their deductions may also take miscellaneous deductions (Impairment-Related Work Expenses) for expenditures such as readers and adapted computer hardware and software.

Deductible medical and dental expenses which exceed 7.5% of an individual's adjusted gross income may include special medications such as insulin and other special items such as guide dogs or other animals used by persons who are visually impaired, blind, or deaf. Contact the Internal Revenue Service (See "ORGANIZATIONS" section below) to obtain publications that explain these benefits, including Publication 907, "Tax Highlights for Persons with Disabilities," Publication 501, "Exemptions, Standard Deduction, and Filing Information," and Publication 524, "Credit for the Elderly or the Disabled." Some states allow extra personal exemptions for legal blindness on state income tax as well.

All states and many local governments have adopted their own laws regarding accessibility. Information about these laws may be obtained from the state or local office serving people with disabilities.

Some lawyers specialize in the legal needs of people with disabilities. Contact the local bar association or a law school for a referral. There are many specialized legal aid organizations that provide services to people with disabilities at no charge or on a sliding fee scale.

The Internet, the computer network supported by the federal government, supplies the text of many federal laws and information about federal programs. Individuals who have a connection to the Internet via their university, workplace, or a commercial online service (such as America Online, Delphi, Compuserve, Prodigy, etc.) may search the information available on the Internet by typing "telnet fedworld.gov" and selecting from the menu.

ORGANIZATIONS

ARCHITECTURAL AND TRANSPORTATION BARRIERS COMPLIANCE BOARD (ATBCB)
1331 F Street, NW, Suite 1000
Washington, DC 20004-1111
(800) 872-2253 (V/TT)   (800) 993-2822 (TT)
(202) 272-5434   (202) 272-5449 (TT)
FAX (202) 272-5447   BBS (202) 272-5448

A federal agency charged with developing standards for accessibility in federal facilities, public accommodations, and transportation facilities as required by the Americans with Disabilities Act and other federal laws. Provides technical assistance, sponsors research, and distributes publications. Publishes a quarterly newsletter, "Access America." All publications available in P, LP, C, PC disk, and B; FREE.

CLEARINGHOUSE ON DISABILITY INFORMATION
Office of Special Education and Rehabilitative Services (OSERS)
Room 3132, Switzer Building
Washington, DC 20202-2524
(202) 205-8241 (V/TT)   (202) 205-8723 (V/TT)

Responds to inquiries about federal legislation and programs for people with disabilities and makes referrals. Publishes newsletter, "OSERS Magazine," FREE.

DISABILITY BUSINESS AND TECHNICAL ASSISTANCE CENTERS
(800) 949-4232 (V/TT)

These federally funded centers located throughout the country provide information on how the Americans with Disabilities Act affects business. FREE materials; P, LP, C, B, and PC disk.

DISABILITY RIGHTS EDUCATION AND DEFENSE FUND (DREDF)
2212 Sixth Street
Berkeley, CA 94710
(800) 466-4232 (V/TT)   (510) 644-2555 (V/TT)
FAX (510) 841-8645

Provides technical assistance, information, and referrals on laws and rights; provides legal representation to people with disabilities in both individual and class action cases; trains law students, parents, and legislators. Publishes "Disability Rights News" monthly; P and C; FREE.

EQUAL EMPLOYMENT OPPORTUNITY COMMISSION (EEOC)

1801 L Street, NW, 10th floor
Washington, DC 20507
(800) 669-3362 to order publications
(800) 669-4000 to speak to an investigator
(800) 800-6820 (TT)
In the Washington, DC metropolitan area, (202) 275-7377
(202) 275-7518 (TT)
FAX (513) 791-2954

Responsible for developing and enforcing regulations for Title I, the employment section of the ADA. Copies of its regulations are available in P, LP, C, computer disk, and B.

INTERNAL REVENUE SERVICE (IRS)

(800) 829-1040   (800) 829-4059 (TT)
telnet fedworld.gov

The IRS provides technical assistance about tax credits and deductions related to accommodations for disabilities. To receive Publication 501, "Exemptions, Standard Deduction, and Filing Information;" Publication 907, "Tax Highlights for Persons with Disabilities;" and Publication 524, "Credit for the Elderly or the Disabled," call (800) 829-3676; (800) 829-4059 (TT). Federal tax forms and publications may be downloaded and printed from the Internet site.

NATIONAL COUNCIL ON DISABILITY (NCOD)
1331 F Street, NW, 10th Floor
Washington, DC 20004
(202) 272-2004   (202) 272-2074 (TT)
FAX (202) 272-2022

An independent federal agency mandated to study and make recommendations about public policy for people with disabilities. Holds regular meetings and hearings in various locations around the country. Publishes newsletter, "Focus;" P, LP, or C; FREE.

OFFICE FOR ELDERLY AND HANDICAPPED PEOPLE
Department of Housing and Urban Development (HUD)
451 7th Street, SW
Washington, DC 20410
(202) 708-2730   FAX (202) 708-1300

Operates programs to make housing accessible, including loan and mortgage insurance for rehabilitation of single or multifamily units. FREE information kit.

OFFICE OF CIVIL RIGHTS
Department of Education
300 C Street, SW
Washington, DC 20202
(202) 205-5413   (800) 358-8247 (TT)
FAX (202) 205-5381

Responsible for enforcing laws and regulations designed to protect the rights of individuals in educational institutions that receive federal financial assistance. Individuals who feel their rights have been violated may file a complaint with one of the ten regional offices.

OFFICE OF CIVIL RIGHTS
Department of Health and Human Services
330 Independence Avenue, SW (Cohen Building)
Washington, DC 20201
(202) 619-0585   FAX (202) 619-3437
(202) 863-0101 (TT)

Responsible for enforcing laws and regulations that protect the rights of individuals seeking medical and social services in institutions that receive federal financial assistance. Individuals who feel their rights have been violated may file a complaint with one of the ten regional offices located throughout the country.

OFFICE OF FEDERAL CONTRACT COMPLIANCE PROGRAMS (OFCCP)
Department of Labor
Employment Standards Administration
200 Constitution Avenue, NW, Room C-3325
Washington, DC 20210
(202) 219-9475   FAX (202) 219-6195

Reviews contractors' affirmative action plans; investigates complaints; and resolves issues between contractors and employees. Ten regional offices serve as liaisons with district offices under their jurisdiction and with the national office.

OFFICE OF TRANSPORTATION REGULATORY AFFAIRS
Department of Transportation
400 Seventh Street, SW
Washington, DC 20590
(202) 366-9305   (202) 755-7687 (TT)

Responsible for developing regulations for transportation of individuals with disabilities required by the Rehabilitation Act and the Americans with Disabilities Act, Titles II and III. Regulations available in P and C.

OFFICE ON THE AMERICANS WITH DISABILITIES ACT
Department of Justice, Civil Rights Division
PO Box 66118
Washington, DC 20035-6118
(800) 514-0301 Information Line
(800) 514-0383 (TT) Information Line
(202) 514-0301   (202) 514-0383 (TT)
BBS (202) 514-6193   telnet fedworld.gov

Responsible for enforcing Titles II and III of the Americans with Disabilities Act. Copies of its regulations are available in P, LP, C, computer disk, B, BBS, and Internet. Callers may request publications, obtain technical assistance, and speak to an ADA specialist.

SOCIAL SECURITY ADMINISTRATION (SSA)
6401 Security Boulevard
Baltimore, MD 21235
(800) 772-1213   (800) 325-0778 (TT)
http://www.ssa.gov/SSA_Home.html/

To apply for Social Security benefits based on disability or Medicare, call the number above to set up an appointment with a Social Security representative, or visit the Social Security office nearest you. The Office of Disability within the Social Security Administration publishes "Social Security Regulations: Rules for Determining Disability and Blindness," FREE.

PUBLICATIONS

AMERICANS WITH DISABILITIES ACT: QUESTIONS AND ANSWERS
Equal Employment Opportunity Commission (EEOC)
1801 L Street, NW, 10th floor
Washington, DC 20507
(800) 669-3362 to order publications
In the Washington, DC metropolitan area, (202) 275-7377
(202) 275-7518 (TT)   FAX (513) 791-2954
BBS (202) 514-6193

This booklet's question and answer format provides explanations of the ADA's effect on employment, state and local governments, and public accommodations. LP, C, B, and through a bulletin board service; FREE.

DIRECTORY OF LEGAL AID AND DEFENDER OFFICES
National Legal Aid and Defender Association
1625 K Street, NW, 8th Floor
Washington, DC 20006
(202) 452-0620

A directory of legal aid offices throughout the U.S. Includes chapters on disability protection/advocacy, health law, and senior citizens. Updated biennially. $30.00

A GUIDE TO LEGAL RIGHTS FOR PEOPLE WITH DISABILITIES
by Marc D. Stolman
Demos Publications
386 Park Avenue South, Suite 201
New York, NY 10016
(800) 532-8663   (212) 683-0072

This book discusses civil rights, insurance, benefits, and legal issues faced by individuals with disabilities. P, C, and disk (DOS or Mac); $19.95, plus $4.00 shipping and handling.

THE MEDICARE HANDBOOK
Social Security Administration
(800) 772-1213   (410) 966-5994

Published annually, this book helps consumers to understand their rights under Medicare, including what it pays for, appeal rights, and where to get additional information. Available in English and Spanish, FREE. Other FREE publications on Medicare are also available. Also available at local Social Security offices.

MEETING THE NEEDS OF EMPLOYEES WITH DISABILITIES
Resources for Rehabilitation
33 Bedford Street, Suite 19A
Lexington, MA 02173
(617) 862-6455   FAX (617) 861-7517

Provides information to help people with disabilities retain or obtain employment. Chapters on vision, mobility, and hearing and speech impairments include information on organizations, products, and services. $42.95 plus $5.00 shipping and handling. See order form on last page of this book.

RED BOOK ON WORK INCENTIVES
A Summary Guide to Social Security and Supplemental Security Income Work Incentives for People with Disabilities
Social Security Administration
(800) 772-1213

Provides an overview of work incentives for individuals who receive SSDI or SSI. Includes impairment-related work expenses, trial work period, continuation of Medicare coverage, earned income exclusion, and other work incentives. LP. Also available at local Social Security offices, FREE.

SUMMARY OF EXISTING LEGISLATION AFFECTING PERSONS WITH DISABILITIES
Office of Special Education and Rehabilitation Services (OSERS)
Clearinghouse on Disability Information
Room 3132, Switzer Building
Washington, DC 20202-2524
(202) 205-8241 (V/TT)   (202) 205-8723 (V/TT)

This book includes sections on income maintenance programs, health, housing, vocational rehabilitation, and transportation; FREE.

TAX OPTIONS AND STRATEGIES: A STATE-BY-STATE GUIDE FOR PERSONS WITH DISABILITIES, SENIOR CITIZENS, VETERANS, AND THEIR FAMILIES
by Bruce E. Bondo
Demos Publications
386 Park Avenue South, Suite 201
New York, NY 10016
(800) 532-8663   (212) 683-0072

Provides information that enables individuals to benefit from federal, state, and local tax provisions such as tax exemptions, credits and/or deductions. $19.95 plus $4.00 shipping and handling.

TAX OPTIONS AND STRATEGIES FOR PEOPLE WITH DISABILITIES
by Steven Mendelsohn
Demos Publications
386 Park Avenue South, Suite 201
New York, NY 10016
(800) 532-8663   (212) 683-0072

This book describes provisions in the tax laws that affect individuals with disabilities, including access to retirement funds to defray disability expenses, deductions available for assistive technology, incentives for employers to hire individuals with disabilities, and dependent care. P, C, and disk (DOS or Mac); $19.95, plus $4.00 shipping and handling.

UNDERSTANDING SOCIAL SECURITY
WORKING WHILE DISABLED... HOW SOCIAL SECURITY CAN HELP
Social Security Administration
(800) 772-1213

These booklets provide basic information about Social Security programs. The Social Security Administration distributes many other titles, including "Disability," "Medicare," "Retirement," "SSI," and "Survivors." Many of these titles are available in LP, B, or C. Also available at local Social Security offices, FREE.

Chapter 3

SELF-HELP GROUPS

Many individuals who have experienced vision loss find that self-help groups are useful before, during, and after formal rehabilitation training. Self-help groups provide both emotional and practical support. The emotional issues discussed may include loss of self-esteem; changing roles in the family; attitudes of friends and family; how to work with physicians to get answers to important medical questions; and how to deal with people in public. Members share practical solutions to common problems such as identifying medication, recording messages, mowing the lawn, and dialing the telephone.

WHERE TO FIND A SELF-HELP GROUP

Physicians or other service providers may provide referrals to self-help groups for people with vision loss. The Community Services section of local telephone directories often lists groups for people with disabilities under "Health and Human Services" or "Disabilities." The "Social Service Organizations" section of the Yellow Pages is also a good source for locating service agencies and information clearinghouses.

Other sources of self-help groups include directories of local agencies in the public library's reference section; staff members at agencies that serve people who are

LIVING WITH LOW VISION: A Resource Guide for People with Sight Loss, Lexington, MA: Resources for Rehabilitation, Copyright 1996

visually impaired or blind; social service or patient education departments of hospitals; and the information and referral service of the local United Way. Self-help groups for people with chronic conditions such as diabetes or multiple sclerosis may discuss vision loss, since it is often a secondary complication.

National self-help clearinghouses, which are centers for information about self-help groups, are listed below. They are good resources for referrals to local self-help groups, literature, and peer counseling training programs. National self-help organizations for individuals who have experienced vision loss are also listed. These organizations have affiliated groups in many areas.

The most recent form of self-help group has evolved as a result of the technological advances in personal computing. Individuals with a personal computer and modem may now dial up a bulletin board service online, where they may exchange information with others who experience the same disabilities or conditions. Chat groups and news groups provide individuals with the opportunity to discuss their insights, offer advice, and ask questions; other individuals respond to their questions and comments.

Some of these groups are available through a direct dial-up to the organization that sponsors the group, while others are available on the Internet or through a subscription to a commercial service (which may also provide access to the Internet). While exchanging information over computer lines is significantly different in character from meeting face-to-face with a group, it provides information and helps to combat social isolation for those in rural areas and those who are unable to leave their homes. It may also serve as a first step in meeting someone with a similar experience who lives in the same geographical area. Notations throughout this book indicate organizations that sponsor news groups or bulletin board services for individuals who are visually impaired or blind.

A variety of formats is available to receive and exchange information. When you join a usenet group, you may read messages and respond to them as well as submit your own information and questions. In order to join a usenet group, your host computer must provide access. When you subscribe to a usenet group, you will automatically receive all new messages whenever you log on. If you decide to exchange messages with just one member, you may send mail directly to that individual's e-mail address.

Listserv enables you to receive information by sending a message to an e-mail address stating you would like to subscribe. You may add your own messages which may in turn generate responses from other members of a group. Protocol requires that you then summarize your responses and mail them to all other members of the listserv group.

STARTING A SELF-HELP GROUP

Many self-help groups are started by individuals with similar conditions or disabilities, while others are started with the help of a professional. Health care professionals are ideally suited to identify and bring together individuals with common problems. A health care provider or rehabilitation counselor may be willing to have a group use his or her office as the site of a first meeting.

Service providers may help to recruit members for a self-help group. Announcements made in publications read by people who are visually impaired or blind, at educational meetings, and on posters on hospital and agency bulletin boards are also good ways to recruit members. At the first meeting, a group coordinator should be selected to arrange for meeting places and times; to locate speakers; and to facilitate group discussions.

Ideally, self-help groups should be in a constant state of evolution, with members leaving as they adapt to their circumstances and new members joining when they are first experiencing vision loss. This changing membership should result in groups with members at various stages of the process; those who have experienced vision loss for a longer period of time will be able to provide advice to those who have just begun to cope with vision loss.

ORGANIZATIONS

The following national clearinghouses and self-help organizations can refer individuals to a self-help group in their area.

AMERICAN SELF-HELP CLEARINGHOUSE
St. Clares-Riverside Medical Center
Denville, NJ 07834
(201) 625-7101   (201) 625-9053 (TT)
FAX (201) 625-8848   CompuServe "Go Good Health"

Provides information and contacts for national self-help groups, information on model groups and individuals who are starting new networks, and state or local self-help clearinghouses. Publishes "The Self-Help Sourcebook," a directory of national and model self-help groups. $9.00

ASSOCIATION FOR MACULAR DISEASES
210 East 64th Street
New York, NY 10021
(212) 605-3719

Membership organization which holds meetings in New York City area; helps to start chapters in other geographical areas; and arranges special programs in other parts of the country. Provides public education, support, and a hot-line for people with macular degeneration. Membership, $20.00, includes newsletter.

CANADIAN COUNCIL ON SOCIAL CONCERN
Self-Help Unit
PO Box 3505, 55 Parkdale Avenue
Ottawa, Ontario K1Y 4G1 Canada
(613) 728-1865   FAX (613) 728-9387

Develops policy on self-help issues, including those related to health. Newsletter, "Initiative: The Self-Help Newsletter," published in English and French, FREE.

FOUNDATION FIGHTING BLINDNESS
1401 Mt. Royal Avenue
Baltimore, MD 21217
(800) 683-5555   (800) 683-5551 (TT)
(410) 225-9400   (410) 225-9409 (TT)
FAX (410) 225-3936

Local chapters, support groups, and information centers for people with retinitis pigmentosa, macular degeneration, and other retinal diseases. Refers individuals with Usher Syndrome to the Usher Syndrome Self-Help Network.

LIGHTHOUSE NATIONAL CENTER FOR VISION AND AGING (NCVA)
111 East 59th Street
New York, NY 10022
(800) 334-5497 (V/TT)   (212) 821-9200
(212) 821-9713 (TT)   FAX (212) 821-9705

Makes referrals to local support groups throughout the

U.S. for adults who are visually impaired or blind. Publishes "Sharing Solutions: A Newsletter for Support Groups," in LP twice a year, FREE.

MACULAR DEGENERATION INTERNATIONAL
2968 West Ina Road, #106
Tucson, AZ 85741
(800) 393-7634   (607) 797-2525
FAX (607) 797-2525

Support network for individuals with early or late onset macular degeneration. Membership, $25.00, includes newsletter and resource guide.

NATIONAL SELF-HELP CLEARINGHOUSE/CUNY
25 West 43rd Street, Room 620
New York, NY 10036
(212) 642-2944

Makes referral to local self-help groups. Quarterly newsletter "Self-Help Reporter," $10.00; and a list of local self-help clearinghouses in the U.S., $1.00.

VISION FOUNDATION, INC.
818 Mt. Auburn Street
Watertown, MA 02172
(617) 926-4232   In MA, (800) 852-3029
FAX (617) 926-1412

Makes referrals to local self-help groups for individuals with vision loss.

PUBLICATIONS AND TAPES

COPING SKILLS

National Library Service for the Blind and Physically Handicapped
1291 Taylor Street, NW
Washington, DC 20542
(800) 424-8567 or 8572 (Reference Section)
(800) 424-9100 (to receive application)
(202) 707-5100   FAX (202) 707-0712

Lists books available on audiocassette and braille that deal with self-esteem, self-development, and shared experiences in coping with life changes, disabilities and chronic conditions. LP, B, and disc; FREE.

DIABETES, VISUAL IMPAIRMENT, AND GROUP SUPPORT: A GUIDEBOOK

by Judith Caditz
The Center for the Partially Sighted
720 Wilshire Boulevard, Suite 200
Santa Monica, CA 90401-1713
(310) 458-3501   FAX (310) 458-8179

This guidebook is designed for individuals with diabetes and vision loss, their families, and the professionals who work with them. Offers suggestions for organizing education/support groups. P and LP, $12.95 plus $2.50 shipping and handling.

A DIRECTORY OF SELF-HELP/MUTUAL AID SUPPORT GROUPS FOR OLDER PEOPLE WITH IMPAIRED VISION
The Lighthouse, Inc.
111 East 59th Street
New York, NY 10022
(800) 334-5497 (V/TT)   (212) 821-9200
(212) 821-9713 (TT)   FAX (212) 821-9705

Lists local support groups throughout the U.S. $10.00

EYE-OPENERS: IDEAS ON HOW TO DEVELOP A SELF-HELP GROUP FOR PERSONS WITH VISION LOSS
by Janet Hirst, Edward Madara, Christina Brino and Sallie Stacey
New Jersey Self-Help Clearinghouse
St. Clare's Riverside Medical Center
Pocono Road
Denville, NJ 07834
(201) 625-7101   (201) 625-9053 (TT)
In NJ, (800) 367-6274

This book provides information about recruiting members, transportation, publicity, running meetings, using professionals, advocacy, and problem solving. LP or C, $10.00.

HELPING YOU HELPS ME
By Karen Hill, revised and updated by Hector Balthazar
Canadian Council on Social Development
PO Box C.P. 3505 Station, 55 Parkdale Avenue
Ottawa, Ontario K1Y 461 Canada
(613) 728-1865   FAX (613) 728-9387

This book provides practical information on starting and maintaining a self-help group. P and C. $8.00, Canadian funds.

PEER COUNSELING: A SMALL GROUP APPROACH
Arkansas Research and Training Center in Vocational Rehabilitation
PO Box 1358
Hot Springs, AR 71902
(501) 624-4411   FAX (501) 624-3515

Offers guidance to novice peer counselors in problem solving, assertiveness, and mutual support. Training package includes a trainer's manual, $6.00; participant's manual, $6.00; and a companion audiocassette, $5.00.

PEER COUNSELING FOR SENIORS
Senior Health and Peer Counseling
2125 Arizona Avenue
Santa Monica, CA 90404-1398
(310) 828-1243   FAX (310) 453-8485

This trainers' guide is designed to help service providers prepare volunteers to conduct peer counseling sessions for older adults. Includes a manual, audiocassettes, and handouts, $375.00. Videotapes on effective training and supervision are also available.

SELF-HELP RESOURCE LIST
VISION Foundation, Inc.
818 Mt. Auburn Street
Watertown, MA 02172
(617) 926-4232   In MA, (800) 852-3029
FAX (617) 926-1412

Lists sources of literature, training materials, and self-help clearinghouses. LP, $5.00

VISION SELF-HELP GROUP MEETING
Resources for Rehabilitation
33 Bedford Street, Suite 19A
Lexington, MA 02173
(617) 862-6455   FAX (617) 861-7517

Audiocassette of a self-help group meeting of people who are visually impaired or blind. $12.00 plus $3.00 shipping and handling.

Chapter 4

READING WITH VISION LOSS

Many options exist to enable individuals with vision loss to continue reading. The alternatives to reading standard print include LARGE PRINT and recorded materials on audiocassette or discs (must be played on NLS slow speed record player). Special radio stations, known as radio reading services, broadcast local newspapers, current books, and magazines. The state agency that serves people who are visually impaired or blind or the local United Way office can direct individuals to services that provide volunteer readers in their area.

Many individuals use magnifiers, closed circuit television reading systems, or reading machines with speech output to continue reading. Specially adapted computer equipment provides access to standard print through the use of scanners and speech output. In addition, books available on CD-ROM are becoming more common. Many CD-ROMs are now multimedia, allowing for graphics, sound, and animation. Because most CD-ROMs are based on the Windows operating system which uses icons, access has been a problem for individuals who are visually impaired or blind. Recently, several manufacturers of adapted software have produced programs that they claim enable people who are visually impaired or blind to use Windows. In addition, Microsoft, the producer of Windows, has announced that Windows 95 will include

LIVING WITH LOW VISION: A Resource Guide for People with Sight Loss, Lexington, MA: Resources for Rehabilitation, Copyright 1996

low vision enhancement features that are installed by default.

Many public libraries have special services for people with vision loss and other disabilities. Libraries often have closed circuit television reading systems, specially adapted computer equipment, and collections of LARGE PRINT books and books on audiocassette. Some libraries have portable versions of adapted equipment that are available on loan to patrons. Many libraries have special outreach or home-bound programs that deliver books to patrons who are unable to get to the library. The reference librarian is a good source for information about the services available for people with vision loss.

In the U.S., individuals who are unable to read standard print because of vision loss or physical limitations which prevent them from holding a book or turning the pages and those with perceptual problems are eligible for services from the National Library Service for the Blind and Physically Handicapped (NLS), 1291 Taylor Street NW, Washington, DC 20542, (800) 424-9100.

A professional service provider must complete an application that indicates the nature of the disability. The NLS provides FREE leisure-time reading materials on audiocassette (playable only on a special 4-track player) and disc (playable only on a special slow speed record player). This special equipment is FREE on loan.

In Canada, special library services for individuals who are blind or visually impaired are provided by the Canadian National Institute for the Blind (CNIB). CNIB provides audiocassette books and magazines, recorded in English and French, to individuals who are visually impaired or blind. National Library Division, 1929 Bayview Avenue, Toronto, Ontario, M4G 3E8 Canada, (416) 480-7520; in Canada, (800) 268-8818.

LARGE PRINT BOOKS

LARGE PRINT books are usually set in 14 point type or larger. 14 point type is more than twice the size of standard newsprint.

This is a sample of 14 point type.
This is a sample of 16 point type.
This is a sample of 18 point type.
This is a sample of 18 point bold type.

The public library is the best source for LARGE PRINT books. "The Complete Directory of Large Print Books and Serials" is published annually by R. R. Bowker and lists all titles available in LARGE PRINT. It should be available in the library's reference section. Most libraries will arrange interlibrary loans of books they do not own.

LARGE PRINT cookbooks, bibles, and reference books are books that readers often want to own rather than borrow. LARGE PRINT books are available in stores and directly from the publishers.

DOUBLEDAY LARGE PRINT HOME LIBRARY
6550 East 30th Street
PO Box 6325
Indianapolis, IN 46206-6325
(800) 688-4442   (317) 541-8920

Hardcover popular fiction and nonfiction, priced the same as standard print books. Minimum number of purchases required. FREE catalogue.

ISIS LARGE PRINT BOOKS
Transaction Publishers
Rutgers - The State University of New Jersey
New Brunswick, NJ 08903
(908) 932-2280   FAX (908) 932-3138

Classic and contemporary literature, self-help, and reference books. FREE catalogue.

LIBRARY REPRODUCTION SERVICE (LRS)
1977 South Los Angeles Street
Los Angeles, CA 90011
(800) 255-5002   (213) 749 2463
FAX (213) 749-8943

Produces LP reproductions of reading materials in 14 to 30 point type on a fee-per-page basis.

RANDOM HOUSE
400 Hahn Road
PO Box 100
Westminster, MD 21157
(800) 733-3000

Fiction and nonfiction titles, crossword puzzle books. 16 point type. FREE catalogue.

READER'S DIGEST LARGE TYPE READER
Reader's Digest Fund for the Blind, Inc.
Box 241
Mount Morris, IL 61054-9982
(800) 877-5293

Selections from Reader's Digest publications, 16 point type. Annual subscription, five volumes; U.S., $9.89; Canada, $12.73.

THORNDIKE PRESS & G.K. HALL LARGE PRINT BOOKS
PO Box 159
Thorndike, ME 04986-0159
(800) 223-6121   FAX (800) 948-2863

Popular fiction and nonfiction, 16 point type. FREE catalogue in LP.

ULVERSCROFT LP BOOKS
PO Box 1230
West Seneca, NY 14224-1230
(800) 955-9659   (716) 674-4270
FAX (716) 674-4195

Classics, contemporary fiction and nonfiction, 16 point type. FREE catalogue.

WHEELER PUBLISHING
PO Box 531
Accord, MA 02018-0531
(800) 588-8881   FAX (617) 871-9173

Fiction and nonfiction bestsellers. 16 point type. FREE catalogue.

TALKING BOOKS

"Talking Books" is the term used to describe books recorded for use by individuals who are unable to read standard print because of vision loss, physical limitations which prevent them from holding a book or turning the pages, or perceptual problems. "Talking Book" cassettes must be played on a special 4-track cassette player. "Talking Book" discs are records which must be played on a special slow speed record player. This equipment is FREE on loan from the National Library Service for the Blind and Physically Handicapped (NLS) in the U.S. or the Canadian National Institute for the Blind in Canada (CNIB). Both organizations also produce many of the recorded books in their collections.

CANADIAN NATIONAL INSTITUTE FOR THE BLIND (CNIB)
National Library Division
1929 Bayview Avenue
Toronto, Ontario, M4G 3E8 Canada
(800) 268-8818   (416) 480-7520
FAX (416) 480-7700   e-mail cnib-library@immedia.ca

NATIONAL LIBRARY SERVICE FOR THE BLIND AND PHYSICALLY HANDICAPPED (NLS)
1291 Taylor Street, NW
Washington, DC 20542
(800) 424-8567 or 8572 (Reference Section)
(800) 424-9100 (to receive application)
(202) 707-5100   FAX (202) 707-0712
telnet marvel.loc.gov (log in as marvel, select Library of Congress Online Systems, select connect to LOCIS, then select "Braille and Audio" for a catalogue of braille and tape publications)

RECORDING FOR THE BLIND AND DYSLEXIC (RFB&D)
20 Roszel Road
Princeton, NJ 08540
(800) 221-4792   (609) 452-0606
FAX (609) 987-8116

Records educational materials on 4-track audiocassette for people who are legally blind or have physical or perceptual disabilities. RFB&D is a major source of recorded textbooks for college students. Requires certification of disability by a medical or educational professional. Charges a one-time registration fee of $37.50. Sells 4-track audiocassette players.

Publishes a catalogue of its recent recordings, "Quarterly Disk Catalog" (QDC), produced on PC or Mac disk, which lists all additions to the RFB&D library during the previous quarter and includes a catalogue of the RFB&D electronic text collection. Subscription, $12.00. Newsletter, "RFB&D

News," P, C, and electronic text; FREE.

VOLUNTEERS WHO PRODUCE BOOKS
National Library Service for the Blind and Physically Handicapped (NLS)
1291 Taylor Street, NW
Washington, DC 10542
(800) 424-8567 or 8572 (Reference Section)
(202) 707-5100   FAX (202) 707-0712

A directory of volunteer groups and individuals in the U.S. who produce LP, C, and B books; FREE.

PERIODICALS

CHOICE MAGAZINE LISTENING
PO Box 10
Port Washington, NY 11050
(516) 883-8280

A bimonthly audio anthology of articles from standard print periodicals. Must be played on a 4-track audiocassette player (see "Talking Books" section, above). FREE

DIALOGUE
c/o Blindskills, Inc.
Box 5181
Salem, OR 97304
(503) 581-4224   FAX (503) 581-1078

Magazine with articles on employment, technology, and

everyday living; includes fiction and poetry by authors who are visually impaired or blind. Published quarterly in LP, 4-track audiocassette, and B. $25.00. Sample copy, $6.00.

MAGAZINES IN SPECIAL MEDIA
National Library Service for the Blind and Physically Handicapped (NLS)
1291 Taylor Street, NW
Washington, DC 20542
(800) 424-8567 or 8572 (Reference Section)
(202) 707-5100   FAX (202) 707-0712

This LARGE PRINT booklet lists the wide variety of magazines which are available FREE in LP, 4-track audiocassette, and disc. FREE

MATILDA ZIEGLER MAGAZINE FOR THE BLIND
80 Eighth Avenue, Room 1304
New York, NY 10011
(212) 242-0263   FAX (212) 633-1601

Magazine available on disc and in braille. Articles from current periodicals as well as information of special interest to individuals who are visually impaired or blind. FREE

NEWSWEEK
American Printing House for the Blind
1839 Frankfort Avenue, PO Box 6085
Louisville, KY 40206-0085
(800) 223-1839   (502) 895-2405
FAX (502) 895-1509

Weekly magazine available on audiocassette (must be played on 4-track audiocassette player); FREE.

NEW YORK TIMES LARGE TYPE WEEKLY
Mail Subscriptions
PO Box 9564
Uniondale, NY 11565-9564
(800) 631-2580   FAX (201) 342-2539

Weekly news summary from the "New York Times." Crossword puzzles included. 16 point type. Subscription, 26 weeks, $35.10; 52 weeks, $70.20.

READER'S DIGEST LARGE-TYPE EDITION
Reader's Digest Fund for the Blind, Inc.
PO Box 241
Mount Morris, IL 61054-9982
(800) 877-5293

Selected articles from the "Reader's Digest," published monthly. U.S., $9.95; Canada, $12.72

RECORDED PERIODICALS
Associated Services for the Blind
919 Walnut Street, 2nd Floor
Philadelphia, PA 19107
(215) 627-0600, extension 208

Subscriptions on 4-track audiocassette for magazines which are not available through the Talking Books Program from the NLS (described above). FREE catalogue.

THE WORLD AT LARGE
PO Box 190330
Brooklyn, NY 11219
(800) 285-2743

Biweekly LARGE PRINT newspaper with articles reprinted from major news magazines. Annual subscription, $39.00.

ELECTRONIC PUBLISHING

A recent advance in publishing is the production of publications in electronic format, using computer disks and CD-ROMs, which are similar to musical compact disks. To date, reference works are the most commonly produced works on CD-ROM, although other types of books are coming on the market in this format as well. Since these publications are used with PCs, they can be accessed by computers that have speech output systems.

THE CD-ROM ADVANTAGE FOR BLIND USERS
National Braille Press
88 St. Stephen Street
Boston, MA 02115
(617) 266-6160   FAX (617) 437-0456

This reference guide describes CD-ROM technology, how it works with speech and braille, and lists titles accessible with braille and speech. P, $15.45; B and disk, $11.95.

FRANKLIN ELECTRONIC PUBLISHERS, INC.
122 Burrs Road
Mt. Holly, NJ 08060
(800) 762-5382   (609) 261-4800
FAX (609) 261-2984

Electronic reference publications with speech output, including English and bilingual dictionaries and thesauruses. FREE catalogue.

RECORDING FOR THE BLIND AND DYSLEXIC (RFB&D)
20 Roszel Road
Princeton, NJ 08540
(800) 221-4792   (609) 452-0606
FAX (609) 987-8116

E-text, RFB&D's collection of electronic books on disk in ASCII text for PCs and Macintosh, includes computer manuals and reference books available for purchase. RFB&D's catalogue, "Quarterly Disk Catalog" (QDC), produced on disk, lists all additions (C and E-text) to the

RFB&D library. $16.00, annual subscription. (See "TALKING BOOKS" section for additional information.)

COMMERCIAL SOURCES OF RECORDED MATERIALS

Bookstores and libraries now carry recorded books on a variety of subjects. These books do not require special playback equipment (unlike the Talking Books listed above); they may be played on standard audiocassette tape players. Often recorded books are abridged versions of the original books. The companies listed below, however, produce unabridged audiocassettes. "Words on Cassette," published annually by R.R. Bowker and available at the reference desk of public libraries, lists commercial sources of books recorded on audiocassette.

BOOKCASSETTE SALES
1810-B Industrial Drive
PO Box 481
Grand Haven, MI 49417
(800) 222-3225   FAX (800) 648-2312

Bestsellers which must be played on stereo tape players. FREE catalogue.

BOOKS ON TAPE
PO Box 7900
Newport Beach, CA 92658
(800) 626-3333   FAX (714) 548-6574

Bestsellers available for rent. FREE catalogue.

CHIVERS AUDIO BOOKS
PO Box 1450
Hampton, NH 03843-1450
(800) 704-2005 FAX (603) 929-3890

Bestsellers available for purchase or rent. FREE catalogue.

RECORDED BOOKS
270 Skipjack Road
Prince Frederick, MD 20678
(800) 638-1304

Fiction and nonfiction titles available for rent. FREE catalogue.

RADIO READING SERVICES

Radio reading services are accessible through special closed channel radio receivers. These services read local newspapers, bestsellers, and special consumer programs. The name and address of a local radio reading service is available from the state agency that provides services to individuals who are visually impaired or blind. Or contact the Association of Radio Reading Services (ARRS), c/o Radio Information Service, 2100 Wharton Street, Suite 140, Pittsburgh, PA 15203 (412) 488-3944. Some state agencies provide receivers to eligible clients; some radio reading services will provide FREE receivers.

RELIGIOUS MATERIALS IN SPECIAL MEDIA

BIBLE ALLIANCE, INC.
PO Box 621
Bradenton, FL 34206
(813) 748-3031   FAX (813) 748-2625

Audiocassettes of the bible and bible studies in English and other languages.   Requires certification of visual impairment by the National Library Service for the Blind and Physically Handicapped or similar organization. FREE.

BIBLES, OTHER SCRIPTURES, LITURGIES AND HYMNALS IN SPECIAL MEDIA
National Library Service for the Blind and Physically Handicapped (NLS)
1291 Taylor Street, NW
Washington, DC 20542
(800) 424-8567 or 8572 (Reference Section)
(202) 707-5100   FAX (202) 707-0712

Reference circular lists religious materials available in special media. P and disc, FREE.

CHRISTIAN RECORD SERVICES
4444 South 52nd Street, Box 6097
Lincoln, NE 68506
(402) 488-0981   (402) 488-1902 (TT)
FAX (402) 488-7582

Publishes religious magazines for bible study in LP, B, and

C. Operates a FREE lending library. FREE catalogue.

DIRECTORY OF RESOURCES FOR THE BLIND AND VISUALLY IMPAIRED
John Milton Society for the Blind
475 Riverside Drive, Room 455
New York, NY 10115
(212) 870-3335

LARGE PRINT directory of religious and secular materials in LP, C, disc, and B; FREE.

JEWISH BRAILLE INSTITUTE
110 East 30th Street
New York, NY 10016
(212) 889-2525

Loans LARGE PRINT English and Hebrew books and recordings in English, Hebrew, Yiddish, and other languages. "JBI Voice" is a monthly audiocassette magazine of Jewish current events and stories. FREE.

SCRIPTURES FOR THOSE WITH SPECIAL NEEDS
American Bible Society
PO Box 5656, Grand Central Station
New York, NY 10164-0851
(800) 322-4253   FAX (212) 408-8765

Bibles available in LP, C, and B. Spanish versions available. FREE catalogue.

WALKER AND COMPANY
435 Hudson Street
New York, NY 10014
(800) 289-2553   (212) 727-8300
FAX (212) 727-0984

Religious titles, biographies, fiction, and nonfiction. FREE catalogue.

MISCELLANEOUS

ASSISTIVE DEVICES FOR READING
National Library Service for the Blind and Physically Handicapped (NLS)
1291 Taylor Street NW
Washington, DC 20542
(800) 424-8567 or 8572 (Reference Section)
(202) 707-5100   FAX (202) 707-0712

Reference circular lists devices that enable individuals with visual or physical disabilities to gain access to information in print. Devices range from magnifiers, page turners, and book holders to computer hardware and software. Products, product evaluations, and vendors are included. LP, FREE.

Chapter 5

HOW TO KEEP WORKING WITH VISION LOSS

One of the greatest fears of individuals with vision loss is that they will be unable to obtain or retain employment. With advances in modern technology, people who are visually impaired or blind are capable of carrying out many job functions that would have been closed to them in the past. It is important that both employers and employees themselves be aware of the simple environmental adaptations and the high tech equipment that can enable individuals who are visually impaired or blind to keep working in their current positions or to enter new positions. Obviously, those individuals with vision loss who are engaged in careers which require excellent vision, such as airplane pilots, truck drivers, and certain medical specialists, require retraining or additional education in order to work in a different field or position.

VOCATIONAL REHABILITATION

Each state has a public agency that provides vocational rehabilitation to individuals who are visually impaired or blind. Vocational rehabilitation services provide retraining, assistance in adapting the work environment, job placement, and in some cases, adaptive equipment. These agencies receive federal funds and must submit a plan to the federal government for approval. Eligibility for

LIVING WITH LOW VISION: A Resource Guide for People with Sight Loss, Lexington, MA: Resources for Rehabilitation, copyright 1996

vocational rehabilitation varies, but most states require that clients be legally blind (See Chapter 1, "EXPERIENCING VISION LOSS," for a definition of legal blindness and more information about rehabilitation services) and there must be a reasonable expectation that vocational rehabilitation will result in job placement. Disability determination must be supported by medical evidence and is decided by the Disability Determination Unit of the vocational rehabilitation agency.

Individuals who are experiencing vision loss but who are not legally blind should not wait for the deterioration of their vision to progress to legal blindness before seeking vocational help. Many types of accommodations can be made to help maintain employment, including adaptive aids, changes in responsibilities and schedules, and trade-offs with other employees. (See Chapter 6, "HIGH TECH AIDS," which describes many adaptive aids.) Vocational rehabilitation services may be obtained from private agencies or practitioners.

Individuals who are eligible for vocational rehabilitation services from a state agency develop an Individualized Written Rehabilitation Plan (IWRP) jointly with a rehabilitation counselor. The IWRP specifies employment goals and the services to be provided by the agency. According to federal law, both the client and the counselor must sign the IWRP, which may be amended or modified with reasonable justification and agreement by both parties.

Vocational rehabilitation services are provided until successful rehabilitation is achieved or until a determination is made that vocational rehabilitation goals cannot be reached. A case may not be closed until the client has been suitably and satisfactorily employed for at least 60 days. The agency's Client Assistance Program (CAP) provides assistance solving any problems encountered in obtaining services.

The Social Security Administration's PASS Program (Plan to Achieve Self Support) provides incentives for people with disabilities to return to work. It allows participants to set aside income and resources for a specific time period while working to achieve an employment oriented goal. These goals may include education, starting a business, or obtaining adaptive equipment. The PASS Program permits participants to collect Supplemental Security Income (SSI) payments during this period. Call the Social Security Administration [(800) 772-1213 or (800) 325-0778 for TT users] to request information on this program.

ENVIRONMENTAL ADAPTATIONS

The work environment may be made accessible for employees who have experienced vision loss, often without great effort or expense. The Americans with Disabilities Act (ADA) requires that employers make reasonable accommodations for individuals with disabilities who are otherwise qualified for the position under consideration (See Chapter 2, "LAWS THAT AFFECT PEOPLE WITH VISION LOSS," for additional information on the ADA).

The workplace should have well-lighted hallways and accessible entries. Elevators should have braille and raised numerals; taped announcements of the floor number are also helpful.

When designing or remodeling an office, the needs of employees who are visually impaired or blind should be a major concern. Contrasting colors should be used for carpeting, furniture, and walls. Placing yellow tape or painting stripes on the edge of steps helps people with visual impairment to navigate. A metal edge on a carpeted step or a change in the texture of the flooring will provide tactile cues for individuals who are blind. Doors should be kept either closed or completely open. Chairs should always be re-positioned under tables or desks. Partially open doors and chairs left in the middle of a room are dangerous to people with vision loss.

Personnel forms and office procedure manuals should be made available in LARGE PRINT, braille, or on audiocassette. Signs should have large letters and good contrast. Telephones may be adapted with LARGE PRINT numerals for use by individuals who are visually impaired. Employees who are totally blind find that raised dots on the 4-5-6 row of a telephone guide them. Similarly, raised dots on the "f" and "j" keys of a keyboard will help when typing. A bold point pen used with bold line paper is a simple suggestion for carrying out everyday writing tasks. Writing guides and signature guides help people to locate lines on a page or to line up their own handwritten lines.

Sometimes increased light or magnification is sufficient to enable employees with visual impairments to perform their jobs; in other instances they may require equipment with LARGE PRINT or speech output.

Some individuals have progressive diseases that may cause their vision to decrease as time passes. Examples of these diseases are retinitis pigmentosa and macular degeneration. These individuals may need to have their work environment modified as their vision deteriorates.

Individuals who are totally blind or who have light perception only will require different types of adaptations than individuals who retain useful vision. These individuals will often use braille to read and write documents, although they use regular computer keyboards as well. Although sighted co-workers are probably unable to read and write braille, computers that are designed to be used with braille also transcribe the data into standard print.

Federal employment opportunities for individuals with disabilities are coordinated by the Office of Personnel Management (See "ORGANIZATIONS" section below) through Federal Job Information Centers located in many states, listed in telephone directories under "U.S. Government." Most jobs are obtained competitively through a combination of written examination and evaluation of education and experience. When necessary, the government provides readers or makes examinations available in braille, LARGE PRINT, or on audiocassette.

Some individuals are given an opportunity to demonstrate their abilities through special appointing techniques called "700-hour trial appointment" or "excepted appointment." Once the individual has successfully completed a trial or served two years in an excepted appointment, his or her job may be noncompetitively converted to a competitive appointment.

ORGANIZATIONS

BREAKING NEW GROUND RESOURCE CENTER
Purdue University
1146 Agricultural Engineering Building
West Lafayette, IN 47907-1146
(800) 825-4264   (317) 494-5088 (V/TT)
FAX (317) 496-1115

Provides assistance to farmers with disabilities in areas such as career decisions, assistive technology, and resources. Publishes "Breaking New Ground" newsletter, in P and C; FREE. Produces "Plowshares Technical Reports," with titles such as "Farming with a Visual Impairment," "Alternative Farm Enterprises for Farmers with Disabilities," and "Rural Public Libraries: A Resource for the Disabled;" $2.00 each.

CAREERS AND TECHNOLOGY INFORMATION BANK (CTIB)
American Foundation for the Blind (AFB)
11 Penn Plaza, Suite 300
New York, NY 10001
(212) 502-7600   FAX (212) 502-7774
Information line (800) 232-5463

Database of individuals who are visually impaired or blind and use assistive technology at work, in school, or at home. Describes jobs, equipment used, training, and how equipment purchase was funded.

CENTER FOR INFORMATION TECHNOLOGY ACCOMMODATIONS (CITA)

General Services Administration (GSA)
Room 2022, KGDO
18th and F Streets, NW
Washington, DC 20405
(202) 501-4906   (202) 501-2010 (TT)
FAX (202) 501-2967   http://www.gsa.gov/coca/

Formerly called the Clearinghouse on Computer Accommodation (COCA), CITA provides federal managers with information about technology for employees with disabilities. Commonly used hardware, software, and workstations are available at a demonstration/resource center at the GSA Central Office, Room 1213. The Internet site provides information about access to technology, including the World Wide Web, legislation, and policy for people with disabilities.

COMPUTER/ELECTRONIC ACCOMMODATIONS PROGRAM (CAP)

Defense Medical Information Management
5109 Leesburg Pike, Suite 810
Falls Church, VA 22041-3206
(703) 756-8812 (V/TT)

Assists Department of Defense in meeting accessibility requirements through information on technology and disability management issues. Publishes "News Bulletin," in LP, disk, and B; FREE.

4-SIGHTS NETWORK
Greater Detroit Society for the Blind
16625 Grand River Avenue
Detroit, MI 48227
(313) 272-3900   FAX (313) 272-6893
BBS (313) 272-7111

A bulletin board service with information on products, rehabilitation, and ADA resources. No user fee other than telephone charges. Log in as "newuser." The "Occupational Information Library for the Blind" provides a vocational information reference guide for employers and potential employees. Lists nearly 500 types of jobs held by people with vision loss, the education and training required, and assistive technology used.

HADLEY SCHOOL FOR THE BLIND
700 Elm Street
Winnetka, IL 60093
(800) 323-4238   In IL, (708) 446-8111
FAX (708) 446-8153

Offers FREE correspondence courses on careers and employment for individuals who are legally blind, have a prognosis of legal blindness, or are hearing impaired with a prognosis of vision loss. Requires ability to read and understand high school level courses. Course catalogue available in LP, C, and B, FREE.

JOB ACCOMMODATION NETWORK (JAN)
918 Chestnut Ridge Road, Suite 1
PO Box 6080
Morgantown, WV 26506-6080
ADA Information, (800) 232-9675
(800) 526-7234 (V/TT)
In Canada, (800) 526-2262 (V/TT)
FAX (304) 293-5407
BBS (800) 342-5526   telnet fedworld.gov

Maintains database of products that facilitate accommodation in the workplace. Provides information to employers about practical accommodations which enable them to employ individuals with disabilities. ADA Information line provides employers with information about compliance with the Americans with Disabilities Act.

JOB OPPORTUNITIES FOR THE BLIND (JOB)
National Federation of the Blind (NFB)
1800 Johnson Street
Baltimore, MD 21230
(800) 638-7518   In MD, (410) 659-9314
FAX (410) 685-5653

A nationwide employment service available to any person who is legally blind and to employers seeking job candidates. Provides literature on job seeking strategies, FREE. Produces "JOB Recorded Bulletin," on audiocassette; FREE.

MAINSTREAM, INC.
3 Bethesda Metro Center, Suite 830
Bethesda, MD 20814
(301) 654-2400 (V/TT)

Provides training and technical assistance, publishes reference guides, and sponsors annual conference to advocate for employment of people with disabilities.

NATIONAL INDUSTRIES FOR THE BLIND (NIB)
524 Hamburg Turnpike, CN969
Wayne, NJ 07474-0969
(201) 595-9200

Conducts a six month internship program for individuals who are legally blind and are seeking professional employment. Requires that candidates have a bachelor's degree in a field related to business or communications and a grade point average of 3.0. Provides stipend, housing, and relocation expenses plus job accommodations. Interns work in one of NIB's offices or industrial facilities.

PRESIDENT'S COMMITTEE ON EMPLOYMENT OF PEOPLE WITH DISABILITIES (PCEPD)
1331 F Street, NW
Washington, DC 20004
(202) 376-6200   (202) 376-6205 (TT)
FAX (202) 376-6219

Advocates on behalf of people with disabilities, holds an annual conference, and sponsors studies. All publications, including "Disability Network News," published three times a year, available in P, C, and B; FREE.

SMALL BUSINESS ADMINISTRATION (SBA)
409 Third Street, SW
Washington, DC 20416
(800) 827-5722

Callers are directed to a menu of messages that provide information about starting a business, financing, counseling and training, SBA services, and other topics.

U.S. OFFICE OF PERSONNEL MANAGEMENT (OPM)
(912) 757-3000   (912) 744-2299 (TT)
BBS (912) 757-3100   telnet fjob.mail.opm.gov

A federal agency that places individuals in civil service positions. Federal Job Information Centers are located throughout the country. Look in the telephone directory under "U.S. Government listings." Information about open examinations and vacancy announcements is available on the Career America Connection on the BBS and telnet sites listed above.

PUBLICATIONS AND TAPES

AMERICAN REHABILITATION
Superintendent of Documents
PO Box 371954
Pittsburgh, PA 15250-7954
(202) 512-1800   FAX (202) 512-2250
telnet federal.bbs.gpo.gov (Port 3001)
BBS (202) 512-1387

Published by the Rehabilitation Services Administration, this magazine provides information on rehabilitation programs, services, and publications. Published quarterly, U.S., $9.00; foreign, $11.25

AMERICANS WITH DISABILITIES ACT HANDBOOK
Superintendent of Documents
PO Box 371954
Pittsburgh, PA 15250-7954
(202) 512-1800   FAX (202) 512-2250
telnet federal.bbs.gpo.gov (Port 3001)
BBS (202) 512-1387

Describes requirements of the Americans with Disabilities Act and provides information on implementation and compliance. $34.00. Also available on the BBS or telnet site.

AMERICANS WITH DISABILITIES ACT: QUESTIONS AND ANSWERS
Consumer Information Center - 5A
PO Box 100
Pueblo, CO 81002

Brochure describes how the ADA applies to employment and places of public accommodation. $1.00 service fee.

BLIND WORKERS
Lions Clubs International, Public Relations Division
300 22nd Street
Oak Brook, IL 60521
(708) 571-5466　　　　　　FAX (708) 571-8890

Videotape describes new technology and training that enable people who are visually impaired or blind to continue working. 23 minutes. $19.95 plus $4.85 shipping and handling.

CAREER PERSPECTIVES: INTERVIEWS WITH BLIND AND VISUALLY IMPAIRED PROFESSIONALS
American Foundation for the Blind (AFB)
c/o American Book Center
Brooklyn Navy Yard, Building No. 3
Brooklyn, NY 11205
(718) 852-9873　　　　　　FAX (718) 935-9647

Twenty professionals discuss their experiences preparing for and obtaining employment. LP, C, and B. $16.95 plus $3.50 shipping and handling.

CAREERS & THE DISABLED
Equal Opportunity Publications
150 Motor Parkway, Suite 420
Hauppauge, NY 11788-5145
(516) 273-0066   FAX (516) 273-8936

Offers career guidance articles and role-model profiles; lists companies seeking qualified job candidates. Published quarterly, $10.00.

THE CAREERS CATALOGUE
Department of Rehabilitation
Canadian National Institute for the Blind (CNIB)
1929 Bayview Avenue
Toronto, Ontario M4G 3E8 Canada
(416) 480-7626   FAX (416) 480-7677

Describes more than 175 jobs in the public and private sectors that are carried out by individuals who are visually impaired or blind. Describes job tasks and job accommodations used. P and C. $19.95, Canadian funds.

CAREERS: JOB SEARCHING AND SUCCESS
National Library for the Blind and Physically Handicapped (NLS)
1291 Taylor Street, NW
Washington, DC 20542
(800) 424-8567 or 8572 (Reference Section)
(202) 707-5100

A bibliography of materials on disc, audiocassette, and

braille that describe career options and job searching skills. Materials listed are available through the NLS regional libraries. FREE.

EMPLOYMENT OF PERSONS WITH PHYSICAL IMPAIRMENTS OR MENTAL RETARDATION IN THE FEDERAL SERVICE
Office of Personnel Management
Washington, DC 20415-0001

Describes federal employment opportunities for individuals with disabilities through competitive appointment or special appointing authorities and special accommodations for examination procedures and on the job. May also be requested from Federal Job Information Centers, listed in the telephone book under "U.S. Government." FREE.

MEETING THE NEEDS OF EMPLOYEES WITH DISABILITIES
Resources for Rehabilitation
33 Bedford Street, Suite 19A
Lexington, MA 02173
(617) 862-6455   FAX (617) 861-7517

Provides information to help people with disabilities retain or obtain employment. Chapters on vision, mobility, and hearing and speech impairments include information on organizations, products, and services. $42.95 plus $5.00 shipping and handling. See order form on last page of this book.

OPENING DOORS: BLIND AND VISUALLY IMPAIRED PEOPLE AND WORK
Department of Rehabilitation
Canadian National Institute for the Blind (CNIB)
1929 Bayview Avenue
Toronto, Ontario M4G 3E8 Canada
(416) 480-7626   FAX (416) 480-7677

Surveys Canadian and international literature on the subject of employment for people with vision loss. P and C. $21.95, Canadian funds.

RED BOOK ON WORK INCENTIVES
A Summary Guide to Social Security and Supplemental Security Income Work Incentives for People with Disabilities
Social Security Administration
(800) 772-1213

Overview of work incentives for individuals who receive SSDI or SSI. Includes impairment-related work expenses, trial work period, continuation of Medicare coverage, earned income exclusion, and other work incentives. Also available from local social security offices. LP, FREE.

TAKE CHARGE: A STRATEGIC GUIDE FOR BLIND JOB SEEKERS
by Rami Rabby and Diane Croft
National Braille Press (NBP)
88 St. Stephen Street
Boston, MA 02115
(617) 266-6160   FAX (617) 437-0456

This book includes examples of the strategies used by successfully employed individuals. P, 4-track audiocassette, PC disk, and B. $19.95 (add $5.00 shipping for print edition).

WORK SIGHT
Braille Institute of America, Inc.
741 North Vermont Avenue
Los Angeles, CA 90029-9988
(800) 272-4553

Individuals who are visually impaired describe their transition to the workplace in this videotape. Emotional and psychological adjustments as well as a team approach to solving problems are discussed. $25.00

WORK SIGHT: VISION AND EMPLOYMENT
The Lighthouse, Inc.
111 East 59th Street
New York, NY 10022
(800) 334-5497 (V/TT)   (212) 821-9200
(212) 821-9713 (TT)   FAX (212) 821-9705

This videotape discusses age-related vision problems in the workplace and recommends environmental adaptations. $25.00, 1/2" or 3/4" format; includes brochures and discussion guide.

Chapter 6

HIGH TECH AIDS

Many people with vision loss use "high tech" electronic aids which have been specially adapted to enhance their remaining vision. These aids include closed circuit television systems (CCTVs) and computers with LARGE PRINT, speech, or braille output. Rapid advances in technology have resulted in the proliferation of a wide variety of such aids. While it is impossible to list all adapted equipment and resources, the major sources are listed below.

Many public libraries and universities have established computer access centers where individuals may see the equipment and have "hands-on" experience before making the investment in their own equipment. Some libraries will lend portable equipment to patrons.

The Technology-Related Assistance for Individuals with Disabilities Act Amendments of 1994 (P.L. 103-218) requires that all states provide detailed information about assistive technology for individuals with disabilities.

FINANCING ADAPTIVE TECHNOLOGY

Adaptive technology is often funded by the state vocational rehabilitation agency as part of the Individualized Written Rehabilitation Plan (IWRP). Some states provide full funding; others provide partial funding.

Vocational rehabilitation services may pay for training to use the equipment and provide job referrals upon completion of training. Employers may also pay for adaptive technology. Community based service organizations such as Lions Clubs may assist individuals in the purchase of adaptive equipment.

If an insurance company is paying for an individual's rehabilitation, the cost of adaptive equipment may be covered by the insurance settlement. The Social Security Administration's PASS Program (described in Chapter 5, "HOW TO KEEP WORKING WITH VISION LOSS") may allow participants to set aside income in order to purchase assistive equipment. The Social Security Administration [(800) 772-1213 or (800) 325-0778 for TT users] will provide information on this program.

PUBLICATIONS, DISKS, AND TAPES

FINANCIAL AID FOR STUDENTS WITH DISABILITIES
HEATH Resource Center
One Dupont Circle, NW, Suite 800
Washington, DC 20036-1193
(800) 544-3284   (202) 939-9320 (V/TT)
FAX (202) 833-4760

Includes information about funding assistive technology.
P, C, and disk (DOS or Mac). Single copy, FREE.

**FINANCIAL AIDS FOR THE DISABLED AND THEIR FAMI-
LIES 1994-1996**
by Gail Ann Schlacter and R. David Weber
Reference Service Press
1100 Industrial Road, Suite 9
San Carlos, CA 94070
(415) 594-0743   FAX (415) 594-0411

A directory of scholarships, fellowships, loans, and awards
for individuals with disabilities. $38.50 plus $4.00
shipping and handling.

TAX HIGHLIGHTS FOR PERSONS WITH DISABILITIES
Publication #907
Internal Revenue Service (IRS)
(800) 829-3676   (800) 829-4059 (TT)

Includes information on taxable and nontaxable income
items. The cost of adaptive equipment may be deductible.

TAX OPTIONS AND STRATEGIES FOR PEOPLE WITH DISABILITIES
by Steven Mendelsohn
Demos Publications
386 Park Avenue South, Suite 201
New York, NY 10016
(800) 532-8663   (212) 683-0072

This book describes provisions in the tax laws that affect individuals with disabilities, including access to retirement funds to defray disability expenses, deductions available for assistive technology, incentives for employers to hire individuals with disabilities, and dependent care. P, C, and disk (DOS or Mac); $19.95, plus $4.00 shipping and handling.

CLOSED CIRCUIT TELEVISION SYSTEMS

Closed Circuit Television Systems (CCTVs) are designed to magnify printed material electronically. The components are a mounted camera, a self-contained light source, a lens that magnifies standard print to various sizes or one fixed to the individual's specifications, and a monitor. Sometimes these systems are called electronic magnifiers. Prices vary by manufacturer and with the size of the monitor.

AMERICAN PRINTING HOUSE FOR THE BLIND

1839 Frankfort Avenue
PO Box 6085
Louisville, KY 40206-0085
(800) 223-1839   (502) 895-2405
FAX (502) 895-1509

Big Picture is a lightweight, portable system which converts a standard black and white or color television set to an electronic magnifier. Includes miniature camera, control box, and A/B switch which allows user to switch back and forth between reading and watching television.

ARTIC TECHNOLOGIES INTERNATIONAL, INC.

55 Park Street, Suite 2
Troy, MI 48083-2753
(810) 588-7370   FAX (810) 588-2650

Produces the MAX Basic, with a black and white monitor.

HUMANWARE, INC.

6245 King Road
Loomis, CA 95650
(800) 722-3393   (916) 652-7253
FAX (916) 652-7296

Produces the ClearView, with 12 or 17 inch black and white or color desktop monitor, and the Viewpoint, which uses a hand held camera to scan material and transmit it to the monitor.

INNOVENTIONS
5921 South Middlefield Road
Littleton, CO 80123-2877
(800) 854-6554   (303) 797-6554

Produces the Magni-Cam, an electronic magnifier that connects to any television set. Magnification depends on television screen size.

MAGNISIGHT
PO Box 2653
Colorado Springs, CO 80901
(800) 753-4767

Produces a variety of black and white and color models. Various screen sizes available. Portable 4 1/2 inch mini-readers and independent cameras to hook up with user's television also available.

OPTELEC
6 Lyberty Way, PO Box 729
Westford, MA 01886
(800) 828-1056   FAX (508) 692-6073

Produces a variety of models, with 14 or 20 inch monitors. Black and white or color options. Magnification of 3X to 60X depending upon model. Passport is a portable video magnifier that provides the field of view of a 14 inch monitor, black and white display, with a maximum of 40x magnification. Operates on AC or rechargeable battery.

OPTEQ
5603 Manatee Avenue West
Bradenton, FL 34209-2543
(813) 795-8932   FAX (813) 761-8306

Models offer black and white or color monitors. 13 to 20 inch monitors available. Also sells i-Trak, a hand held CCTV that may be used with any television set; magnification varies depending on TV screen size.

TELESENSORY
455 North Bernardo Avenue, PO Box 7455
Mountain View, CA 94039-7455
(800) 227-8418   (415) 960-0920
FAX (415) 969-9064

Produces a variety of monitor sizes, including 14 inch, 19 inch, and hand held models and a choice of black and white or color displays. Enhanced models may be used with personal computer monitors. Demonstration video, "See for Yourself," FREE. Newsletter, "In Focus," is published in P and disk; FREE.

COMPUTERS

The rapid growth in computer technology has resulted in increased options for individuals who have experienced vision loss. Some standard computers on the market are equipped with features that enable users to magnify print size on the screen a specified number of times. For example, the Macintosh includes a standard feature called Close View, which enables the user to magnify text on the screen. The popular operating system "Windows," when used in conjunction with appropriate word processing software, allows selection of font sizes on the screen. Access to Windows has been somewhat limited for individuals who are visually impaired or blind, because the system relies heavily on graphics which speech output systems have been unable to handle. Some software manufacturers claim that they have successfully overcome these problems. Microsoft, the producer of Windows, has announced that low vision enhancements will be installed by default in Windows 95.

Some software packages increase the size of print on the screen of PCs and Macintosh computers. In addition, large monitors, while usually more expensive than standard monitors, may enlarge print size sufficiently to enable some people with vision loss to continue using a standard computer.

Synthetic speech screen access used along with a magnification system reinforces what is displayed on the screen, reduces fatigue, and often allows the use of less magnification and a greater field of view. Pitch, rate, volume, and intonation of the synthetic voice should be considered when choosing a particular speech synthesizer.

A significant addition to assistive technology for individuals who are visually impaired or blind is the optical character reader, which scans printed material and converts it to a machine-readable format that can be produced in speech or braille. Optical character readers are used in conjunction with character recognition software.

Several bulletin board services offer information in the latest technology, job openings, and meetings of computer users who are visually impaired or blind. Individuals may access these bulletin boards with the use of a modem and a specially adapted computer, receiving the data in LARGE PRINT, speech, or braille.

It is wise to explore the various options and then make a decision based both on cost and which options are right for the specific situation. In some instances, vocational rehabilitation professionals, job placement specialists, low vision specialists, or staff from special computer centers for people with vision loss may visit the home or workplace, assess individual needs, and demonstrate the options that will serve best. (See Chapter 5, "HOW TO KEEP WORKING WITH VISION LOSS.")

ORGANIZATIONS

CANADIAN NATIONAL INSTITUTE FOR THE BLIND (CNIB)
Technical Aids Service
1929 Bayview Avenue
Toronto, Ontario M4G 3E8 Canada
(416) 486-2636   FAX (416) 480-7677

Provides consultation and demonstration of high and low tech products and facilitates funding for purchase and maintenance of equipment.

CENTER FOR SPECIAL EDUCATION TECHNOLOGY
Council for Exceptional Children
1920 Association Drive
Reston, VA 22091-1589
(703) 620-3660 (V/TT)   FAX (703) 264-9494

Collects and exchanges information about the use of technology in the education of children and youth with disabilities.

FOUNDATION FOR TECHNOLOGY ACCESS
2173 East Francisco Boulevard, Suite 1
San Rafael, CA 94901
(415) 455-4575

Operates Alliance Technology Resource Centers which provide access to assistive technology for individuals with disabilities. Services include information and resources, workshops, user groups, technical support, and hands-on demonstrations. Centers are located in many states and Canada.

NATIONAL CRISTINA FOUNDATION
591 West Putnam Avenue
Greenwich, CT 06830
(203) 622-6000   FAX (203) 622-6270

Distributes donations of surplus or obsolete computer hardware or software to organizations or individuals with disabilities.

TECHNOLOGY CENTER
American Foundation for the Blind (AFB)
11 Penn Plaza, Suite 300
New York, NY 10001
(212) 502-7600   FAX (212) 502-7774
Information line (800) 232-5463
In New York state, (212) 502-7657

Develops and adapts consumer products with speech or tactile output. Evaluations of high tech products conducted by consumers and Center staff are published in "Random Access," a column in "Journal of Visual Impairment and Blindness" (JVIB). JVIB is available at many university libraries.

TRACE RESEARCH AND DEVELOPMENT CENTER ON COMMUNICATION, CONTROL AND COMPUTER ACCESS FOR HANDICAPPED INDIVIDUALS
S-151 Waisman Center
University of Wisconsin-Madison
1500 Highland Avenue
Madison, WI 53705-2280
(608) 263-2309   (608) 263-5408 (TT)

Offers workshops in computer access for people with disabilities and a wide variety of publications on computer accessibility. FREE catalogue.

ADAPTIVE TECHNOLOGIES FOR LEARNING & WORK ENVIRONMENTS
by Joseph J. Lazzaro
Customer Service
American Library Association
155 North Wacker Drive
Chicago, IL 60606
(800) 545-2433

This book explores adaptive technology designed for use by individuals with disabilities, including blindness and visual impairment, deafness and hearing impairment, and motor and/or speech impairments. It focuses on personal computer hardware and software and applications such as computer networks, online services and bulletin boards, and CD-ROM. It also lists funding sources, training and technical support resources, and equipment vendors. $45.00 plus $6.00 shipping and handling. Also available on audiocassette on loan from National Library Service for the Blind and Physically Handicapped regional libraries, RC 37741.

CLOSING THE GAP
PO Box 68
Henderson, MN 56044
(612) 248-3294   FAX (612) 248-3810

This bimonthly newsletter reviews hardware and software products developed for users with disabilities. U.S.,

$29.00; Canada and Mexico, $44.00; other countries, $60.00. Annual hardware and software directory published as February/March issue. The organization also provides training and consulting services and holds an annual conference.

COMPUTER RESOURCES FOR PEOPLE WITH DISABILITIES
by The Alliance for Technology Access
Hunter House
PO Box 2914
Alameda, CA 94501
(800) 266-5592   FAX (510) 865-4295

This book guides readers in making decisions based on personal goals and resources related to assistive technology. Includes resource list of organizations and vendors. $14.95

THE HANDBOOK OF ASSISTIVE TECHNOLOGY
by Gregory Church and Sharon Glennen
Singular Publishing Group, Inc.
4284 41st Street
San Diego, CA 92015
(800) 521-8545   FAX (800) 774-8398

Provides an overview of funding; adaptive access including LARGE PRINT, speech, and braille. Suggestions for integrating assistive technology in the community and classroom. Product directory. $39.95

THE LARGE PRINT COMPUTER DICTIONARY
by Donald D. Spencer
Camelot Publishing Company
PO Box 1357
Ormond Beach, FL 32175
(904) 672-5672

Defines 1200 popular computer terms. $24.95

NATIONAL BRAILLE PRESS
88 St. Stephen Street
Boston, MA 02115
(617) 266-6160   FAX (617) 437-0456

Publishes computer tutorials for word processing and database programs, spreadsheets, and CD-ROM in various formats, including P, C, disk, and B. FREE catalogue.

RECORDED PERIODICALS
Associated Services for the Blind
919 Walnut Street, 2nd Floor
Philadelphia, PA 19107
(215) 627-0600, extension 208

Subscriptions on 4-track audiocassette for popular computer magazines such as "Computers," "Computerworld," and "Macuser" which are not available in special media elsewhere. FREE price list.

SOLUTIONS: ACCESS TECHNOLOGIES FOR PEOPLE WHO ARE BLIND

by Olga Espinola and Diane Croft
National Braille Press (NBP)
88 St. Stephen Street
Boston, MA 02115
(617) 266-6160   FAX (617) 437-0456

Describes adaptive computer devices, bulletin boards, and publications. Includes interviews with individuals who train others to use adaptive devices. P, 4-track audiocassette, and PC disk. $21.95. Add $5.00 shipping and handling for standard print edition.

TECHNOLOGY UPDATE

Sensory Access Foundation
385 Sherman Avenue, Suite 2
Palo Alto, CA 94306
(415) 329-0430   FAX (415) 323-1062

A newsletter that describes recent developments in technology for users who are visually impaired or blind. P, LP, C, and PC disk. Individuals in the U.S. who are visually impaired, $30.00; foreign, $47.00; other individuals, U.S., $37.00; foreign, $57.00; organizations, U.S., $47.00; foreign, $67.00.

CARROLL CENTER FOR THE BLIND
Computer Services
770 Centre Street
Newton, MA 02158
(617) 969-6200   (800) 852-3131
FAX (617) 969-6204

Offers evaluation and training in use of LARGE PRINT, speech, and braille output equipment. Tuition fees vary according to eligibility for a variety of subsidy funding sources. Housing available.

COMPUTER CENTER FOR THE VISUALLY IMPAIRED
Baruch College
17 Lexington Avenue, Box H0648
New York, NY 10010
(212) 802-2148

Provides training courses in personal computers and software programs; career counseling; and an introductory adaptive computing course for parents and professionals.

HADLEY SCHOOL FOR THE BLIND
700 Elm Street
Winnetka, IL 60093
(800) 323-4238   In IL, (708) 446-8111
FAX (708) 446-8153

Offers FREE correspondence courses on microcomputers

and word processing for individuals who are legally blind, have a prognosis of legal blindness, or are hearing impaired with a prognosis of vision loss. Requires ability to read at the high school level. Course catalogue available in LP, C, and B; FREE.

LIONS WORLD SERVICES FOR THE BLIND
2811 Fair Park Boulevard
PO Box 4055
Little Rock, AR 72214
(501) 664-7100   FAX (501) 664-2743

Offers courses in computer programming, word processing, and other software packages. Housing available.

STORER COMPUTER ACCESS CENTER
Sight Center, Cleveland Society for the Blind
1909 East 101st Street
Cleveland, OH 44106
(216) 791-8118   FAX (216) 791-1101

Evaluation and training center for use of LARGE PRINT, speech, and braille computer access devices. Short term rental of equipment. Housing available.

UNIVERSITY OF NEW ORLEANS TRAINING AND RESOURCE CENTER FOR THE BLIND
ADC 40, Lakefront-East Campus
New Orleans, LA 70148
(504) 286-7096   (504) 286-7431 (TT)
FAX (504) 286-7294

Academic year and summer continuing education courses in word processing, database management, medical transcription, and Lotus. Career counseling available.

ADAPTED COMPUTER HARDWARE, SOFTWARE, AND ACCESSORIES

Ai SQUARED
PO Box 669
Manchester Center, VT 05255-0669
(802) 362-3612   FAX (802) 362-1670

Produces ZoomText, LARGE PRINT software for PCs with graphics magnification, DOS or Windows interface, and font editor. inFocus is a memory resident program with 2X magnification for text and graphics. Visability is a software program, used with a PC and scanner, that produces magnified text.

AMERICAN PRINTING HOUSE FOR THE BLIND (APH)
APH Microcomputer Division
1839 Frankfort Avenue, PO Box 6085
Louisville, KY 40206-0085
(800) 223-1839   (502) 895-2405
FAX (502) 895-1509

Sells adaptive computer hardware and software and computer manuals for Apple products in LP, C, and B. Publishes newsletter, "Micro Materials Update," in LP and C; FREE.

APPLE COMPUTER, INC.
Office of Special Education Programs
One Infinite Loop
Cupertino, CA 95014
(800) 776-2333   (800) 833-6223 (TT)
FAX (800) 462-4396

Offers a packet of information which describes accessibility features for users of Macintosh and Apple II equipment; includes Macintosh Disability Resources (MDR), a database of access products on disk; FREE. Offers "eWorld," an online information service that includes databases, bulletin boards, chat rooms, discussion forums, and software libraries. Call (800) 775-4556 for starter kit or write: eWorld Starter Kit, Apple Computer, Inc., PO Box 4493, Bridgeton, MO 63044-9718.

ARKENSTONE
1390 Borregas Avenue
Sunnyvale, CA 94089
(800) 444-4443   (800) 833-2753 (TT)
(408) 752-2200   FAX (408) 745-6739

Produces An Open Book, designed for individuals without personal computer skills, which scans text and converts it to speech. Open Book Unbound software used with a scanner and speech synthesizer provides speech access to a PC. Available in versions that read more than one dozen languages. First Reader Program offers reconditioned products at discount.

ARTIC TECHNOLOGIES INTERNATIONAL, INC.
55 Park Street, Suite 2
Troy, MI 48083-2753
(810) 588-7370   FAX (810) 588-2650

Produces screen enlargers, speech synthesizers, and screen access systems including hardware, software, tutorials, and accessories. "Visions Newsletter" published three times a year.

BERKELEY SYSTEMS, INC.
2095 Rose Street
Berkeley, CA 94709
(510) 540-5535   (510) 540-0709 (TT)
FAX (510) 540-5115

outSPOKEN uses the Macintosh's built in speech synthesizer to make word processing programs, spreadsheets, and databases accessible to blind users.

BLAZIE ENGINEERING
109 East Jarrettsville Road, Unit D
Forest Hill, MD 21050
(410) 893-9333   FAX (410) 836-5040

Produces the Braille 'n Speak, a portable talking braille notetaker, which has additional features such as a talking clock and calendar, calculator, and stopwatch. May be used with a computer terminal and a modem. Battery powered speech synthesizer.

DECtalk
Digital Equipment Corporation
Two Penn Plaza
New York, NY 10121
(212) 856-3100

Text-to-speech system converts standard ASCII text to a human quality voice. The speech type and rate are adjustable. Special prices for individuals who are visually impaired or blind.

EYE RELIEF
Ski Soft Publishing
1644 Massachusetts Avenue, Suite 79
Lexington, MA 02173
(800) 662-3622   (617) 863-1876
FAX (617) 861-0086

Designed for PCs, this word processing program offers six sizes of on-screen type, oversized cursor, wordwrap scrolling, and LP manual.

GW MICRO
310 Racquet Drive
Fort Wayne, IN 46825
(219) 482-3625   FAX (219) 482-2492

Produces Sounding Board, an internal speech synthesizer for PCs. Produces Vocal-Eyes, a screen review reader to be used in conjunction with speech synthesizer. SPEAK OUT is a portable, battery powered speech synthesizer.

Instruction manuals available in LP, C, and disk. Also sells other computer systems, synthesizers, software, and accessories. Newsletter, "Voice of Vision," published quarterly in LP, C, PC disk, and B.

HUMANWARE, INC.
6245 King Road
Loomis, CA 95650
(916) 652-7253   FAX (916) 652-7296

Produces computers with speech, LARGE PRINT, or braille output and Speakwriter, a talking typewriter. Keynote GOLD speech synthesizer with MasterTouch screen reading software. Available in English, French, and Spanish. The Keynote Companion is a palmtop device with speech output for applications such as a word processor, spell checker, calculator, and calendar.

IBM INDEPENDENCE SERIES
PO Box 1328
Boca Raton, FL 33429-1328
(800) 426-4832   (800) 426-4833 (TT)
In Canada, (800) 465-7999

Screen Magnifier/2 enlarges text and images up to 32 times. Screen Reader/2 produces speech output of screen text; provides speech output of IBM's Graphical User Interface (GUI). Screen Reader/DOS produces speech output and interfaces with enlargement software.

JAWS (Job Access With Speech)
Henter-Joyce
2100 62nd Avenue North
St. Petersburg, FL 33702-7142
(800) 336-5658   (813) 576-5658
FAX (813) 528-8901

A screen access software program to use with a variety of speech synthesizers designed for PCs. Also sells instructional tapes for using WordPerfect and DOS with JAWS.

KIDSVIEW SOFTWARE, INC.
PO Box 98
Warner, NH 03278
(800) 542-7501   (603) 927-4428

Specializes in LARGE PRINT software for Apple II, PC/MS-DOS, and Commodore 64 computers. Also sells Kidsword, a LARGE PRINT word processor.

MENTOR O & O INC.
3000 Longwater Drive
Norwell, MA 02061-1672
(800) 992-7557   (617) 871-6950
FAX (617) 871-7785

Sells the Horizon Low Vision Magnifier, a digital scanner that converts text to a single line which scrolls across a 14 inch monitor. Up to 35X magnification.

MICROSYSTEMS SOFTWARE, INC.
600 Worcester Road
Framingham, MA 01701
(800) 828-2600   (508) 879-9000
FAX (508) 626-8515

Produces MAGic, 2X screen magnification software for DOS and Windows, and MAGic Deluxe, up to 12X magnification. LP user guide available for MAGic Deluxe. Demonstration copy of MAGic Deluxe available by downloading from the Microsystems Software bulletin board, (508) 875-8009.

OPTELEC
6 Lyberty Way, PO Box 729
Westford, MA 01886
(800) 828-1056   In MA, (508) 392-0707
FAX (508) 692-6073

LARGE PRINT software which operates on any PC. Compatible with speech packages, enabling the user to have speech back-up while using LARGE PRINT software. LP-DOS Version 5.0 supports Microsoft Windows.

TELESENSORY
455 North Bernardo Avenue, PO Box 7455
Mountain View, CA 94039-7455
(800) 227-8418   (415) 960-0920
FAX (415) 969-9064

Produces hardware and software with LARGE PRINT and

speech output; an optical scanner designed to be used with LARGE PRINT, speech, and braille systems; and many other computer products for people who use braille.

XEROX IMAGING SYSTEMS
9 Centennial Drive
Peabody, MA 01960
(800) 421-7323   (508) 977-2000
FAX (617) 977-2148

The Reading Edge uses a scanner, speech synthesizer, and software to read printed material in a choice of speaking voices. Includes headphone and tape recorder jacks as well as serial port for linking to computer.

MISCELLANEOUS

There are several devices which may provide the magnification or contrast needed to continue using a standard computer system.

Contrast enhancement filters attach to the computer monitor, increase contrast, and reduce glare from natural and overhead light sources. Visor-like hoods will also shield the monitor from overhead lighting. Local computer supply stores are the best source for these products.

Asymmetric lighting illuminates the work area without glare. Asymmetric lighting is available in desk top models, on flexible arms which may be surface or wall mounted or used with a floor stand. Glare may also be reduced by removing a light bulb or two from an overhead fixture and using a desk lamp to focus on work material.

Louvers are available for some lamps to further reduce glare.

CompuLenz, which fits on most computer monitors, enlarges character size while eliminating distortion and light reflection. Available from Florida New Concepts Marketing, PO Box 261, Port Richey, FL 34673-0261, (800) 456-7097.

Self-adhesive keyboard labels with 38 point letters and 32 point numbers are available in black print on yellow or white print on black. Braille keytop labels and home-row indicators are also available. Order from Hooleon Corporation, PO Box 230, Cornville, AZ 86325, (800) 937-1337 or (602) 634-7515

Typing stands or document holders placed beside or attached to the computer or monitor reduce head and neck movement. Document holders which have flexible arms allow the computer user to move material closer, a useful feature for individuals using low vision aids.

Chapter 7

MAKING EVERYDAY LIVING EASIER

Adapting to vision loss often requires advance planning for everyday activities as well as for travel. People with vision loss should not hesitate to ask for help and directions when in an unfamiliar place. Most people will be glad to help when they understand the individual's needs. Sometimes people are overly solicitous or protective; in such situations, individuals should not hesitate to state what type of help is required, if any.

Individuals who have mobility problems should consider taking orientation and mobility (O and M) lessons from an instructor at a public or private agency or from a private practitioner. The O and M instructor teaches skills in orientation to familiar places and safe travel techniques. Instruction on how to use a cane or a referral to a service that trains guide dogs may also be provided. Choosing a cane or a guide dog is an extremely personal decision and should be made only after obtaining information about the advantages and disadvantages of each.

ENVIRONMENTAL ADAPTATIONS AND HOUSING

Individuals with vision loss do not usually require structural changes to their living environment but instead will use hearing, smell, and touch to augment their vision

LIVING WITH LOW VISION: A Resource Guide for People with Sight Loss, Lexington, MA: Resources for Rehabilitation, Copyright 1996

for orientation and daily living activities. The need for environmental modifications depends upon the individual's degree of visual impairment and other disabilities. Good lighting, signs with large letters and good contrast, and clear aisles are just a few examples of adaptations that make people with vision loss more comfortable.

Other inexpensive environmental modifications and ordinary appliances include:

- Increased illumination on the exterior and interior of the house. Timers are useful for returning home after dark.
- High contrast tape or paint used to mark thresholds and the edges of steps.
- Elevator control buttons with raised characters and braille symbols. These markings should also be on the elevator door-frame on each floor to confirm the destination.
- Cabinets with sliding doors to reduce the danger of bumping into conventional doors left open.
- Appliances such as microwave ovens and hot water dispensers that make meal preparation easier.

Individuals with vision loss may find that increased lighting helps significantly. Fluorescent lighting diffuses evenly and is inexpensive, but it produces less contrast, may flicker, and is harsh. Diffusing filters may solve these problems. The incandescent light of a standard bulb offers more contrast and can be directed, but it produces shadows and glare. Diffusers and additional lighting spread the light and reduce shadows. A combination is often the best choice; fluorescent for general lighting, incandescent for near tasks. Halogen bulbs emit a whiter light than incandescent bulbs, making reading easier; last longer; and produce more light per watt. Dimmer switches help control glare from indoor lights. Glasses with glare control lenses are helpful outdoors.

A combination of light and dark colors in interior decorating and for kitchen utensils and serving pieces allows differentiation between objects. For example, it is difficult to see a piece of steak on a brown plate, but placing a steak on a white plate makes it more visible. When painting the interior of a house, contrasting colors should be used for walls and stairs. Stove and thermostat dials should be marked at commonly used settings with nail polish or a similar type of material. It is crucial to replace household items and clothing in the same locations and to ask household members to do the same. Halls should be kept clear and nonskid flooring should be used whenever possible.

Rehabilitation teachers and occupational therapists who have had professional training to work with individuals who are visually impaired or blind conduct functional assessments and provide individualized instruction in activities of daily living. They can offer many suggestions for appropriate environmental adaptations.

INGENIOUS AIDS AND DEVICES

There are many useful aids and devices, ranging from the simple to complex, which help people with vision loss to live independently. Many agencies that provide services to people with vision loss have stores that sell common aids and devices. Often people find that the devices they develop for themselves are the most useful, as they are specifically designed for their own lifestyles.

Magnifiers are helpful in many situations. There are many different types of magnifiers available for different tasks. For example, a pocket magnifier is useful for shopping. Magnifiers that hang from the neck leave the hands free for sewing or other manual tasks.

A bold felt tip pen kept near the telephone is very useful when taking messages. LARGE PRINT letters on self-adhesive tape, raised dots, and special glues are useful for labeling items such as canned goods, medications, and dials on appliances. Recreational items such as playing cards, bingo cards, and crossword puzzle books are available in LARGE PRINT. LARGE PRINT or tactile watches and "talking" watches, clocks, thermometers, and blood sugar monitors are other useful devices.

Businesses are able to make activities easier by providing information on audiocassette or in LARGE PRINT. For example, some banks provide bank account information on audiocassette and offer LARGE PRINT checks for sale.

Television is more accessible to people with vision loss through Descriptive Video Service (DVS), which uses an additional channel to narrate a description of the actions and settings that take place in the program. It is accessible through a stereo television or a stereo VCR that includes the Second Audio Program (SAP) feature, or an SAP receiver, which is a special stereo attachment for a television. At present, DVS is available on a small portion of public broadcasting's program schedule. The local public broadcasting station can provide information about its DVS programming. In some areas, the DVS narration is broadcast over the local radio reading service.

Narrative Television Network (NTN) produces talk shows and describes movie classics which are broadcast four hours per week on cable systems nationwide. Free to cable operators and stations, it does not require the purchase of additional equipment. The narration is part of the main sound channel, not transmitted on a separate SAP channel. Individuals should contact their local cable system to inquire whether it carries NTN.

ABLEDATA

National Rehabilitation Information Center (NARIC)
8455 Colesville Road, Suite 935
Silver Spring, MD 20910-3319
(800) 227-0216   (301) 588-9284
BBS (301) 589-3563
telnet fedworld.gov (select 8, then 1, then 115; ABLEDATA information is available in the "files" area.)

A database of products for personal care, recreation, and transportation. First 20 items from database search, FREE; a fee is charged for longer searches. Also available on CD-ROM, $25.00; monthly update files, $25.00 per release cycle (four updates). Information from ABLEDATA is available from ABLE INFORM, which NARIC operates at the telnet address above. FREE.

AUDIOVISION

416 Holladay Avenue
San Francisco, CA 94110
(415) 641-4589

Provides descriptive narrative of art exhibits, television, plays, and other media. Provides training to individuals and organizations in methods of adding descriptive narration.

BARRIER-FREE DESIGN CENTRE
College Park, 444 Yonge Street
Toronto, Ontario M5B 2H4 Canada
(416) 977-5010   (416) 977-5225 (TT)
FAX (416) 977-5264

Provides education, information, and technical consultation in barrier-free design and construction for Canadians with disabilities. Publishes professional guides for barrier-free design.

CENTER FOR ACCESSIBLE HOUSING
North Carolina State University
Box 8613
Raleigh, NC 27695-8613
(919) 737-3082 (V/TT)

A federally funded research and training center that works toward improving housing for people with disabilities. Provides technical assistance, training, and publications. Publishes newsletter, "News," P, LP, C, and disk; FREE.

DESCRIPTIVE VIDEO SERVICE (DVS)
WGBH
125 Western Avenue
Boston, MA 02134
(617) 492-2777, extension 3490

The national DVS broadcast service through which public broadcasting stations receive DVS programs. DVS maintains a list of the local public broadcasting stations that carry DVS programming. Can advise individuals where they may purchase SAP TV receivers. Publishes "DVS Guide," in LP, C, and B; FREE. Sells DVS videotapes of popular movies; call (800) 736-3099 for FREE catalogue.

AIDS FOR EVERYDAY LIVING WITH VISION LOSS
Resources for Rehabilitation
33 Bedford Street, Suite 19A
Lexington, MA 02173
(617) 862-6455   FAX (617) 861-7517

A LARGE PRINT (18 point bold type) publication that describes vendors of aids that help people with vision loss remain independent. Minimum purchase, 25 copies. $1.25 per copy plus shipping and handling. Discounts available for purchases of 100 or more copies. See order form on last page of this book.

THE DO-ABLE RENEWABLE HOME
by John P. S. Salmen
American Association of Retired Persons (AARP)
Consumer Affairs-Program Department
601 E Street, NW
Washington, DC 20049
(202) 434-2277

Describes how individuals with disabilities can modify their homes for independent living. Room by room modifications are accompanied by illustrations. FREE.

GUIDE TO GUIDE DOG SCHOOLS
by Ed and Toni Eames
Disabled on the Go
3376 North Wishon
Fresno, CA 93704-4832
(209) 224-0544

This guide provides information for individuals considering use of a guide dog and describes 14 guide dog training programs in the U.S. and two in Canada. P and computer disk, $10.00. Also available on audiocassette on loan from National Library Service for the Blind and Physically Handicapped regional libraries, RC 38777.

HOME SAFETY CHECKLIST FOR OLDER CONSUMERS
U.S. Consumer Product Safety Commission
Washington, DC 20207
(800) 638-2772

Provides information on simple, inexpensive repairs and safety recommendations. Single copy, FREE. Available in English and Spanish.

HOUSING AND SUPPORT SERVICES FOR PHYSICALLY DISABLED PERSONS IN CANADA
Canadian Rehabilitation Council for the Disabled (CRCD)
45 Sheppard Avenue East, Suite 801
Toronto, Ontario M2N 5W9 Canada
(416) 250-7490 (V/TT)   FAX (416) 229-1371

Lists accessible housing options and other support

services for people who live in Canada. Available in English and French. Members, $20.00; nonmembers, $26.00; plus $3.00 shipping and handling, Canadian funds.

INDEPENDENT LIVING
Public Affairs Directorate
Health & Welfare Canada
Disabled Persons Unit
Ottawa, Ontario K1A 1B5 Canada

A series of pamphlets on independent living; includes food preparation, appliances, reaching aids, bathroom equipment and bathing aids, and lifting aids; FREE.

MAKING LIFE MORE LIVABLE
by Irving R. Dickman
American Foundation for the Blind (AFB)
c/o American Book Center
Brooklyn Navy Yard, Building No. 3
Brooklyn, NY 11205
(718) 852-9873   FAX (718) 935-9647

This LP guide uses pictures to demonstrate many adapted aids. $16.95 plus $3.50 postage and handling. Also available FREE on loan on 4-track audiocassette from the National Library Service, RC 22319.

A STREET TO SHARE
Foundation Centre Louis-Hebert
525 boulevarde Hamel Est, aile J
Quebec, Quebec G1M 2S8 Canada
(418) 529-6991

This videotape presents typical situations experienced by individuals who are visually impaired or blind as they travel in their community. Makes suggestions for efficient and effective assistance. $28.00, U.S. funds.

TOOLS FOR INDEPENDENT LIVING and DESIGNS FOR INDEPENDENT LIVING
Appliance Information Service (AIS)
Whirlpool Corporation
Administrative Center
Benton Harbor, MI 49022

Provide information on adaptations for major appliances such as control panel overlays, large graphics, and over-sized pushbuttons. Also provides use and care manuals and cookbooks in LP, C, and B; FREE.

WHATEVER WORKS: CONFIDENT LIVING FOR PEOPLE WITH IMPAIRED VISION
by Nancy Paskin and Lisa Anne Soucy-Moloney
The Lighthouse, Inc.
111 East 59th Street
New York, NY 10022
(800) 334-5497 (V/TT)   (212) 821-9200
(212) 821-9713 (TT)   FAX (212) 821-9705

Provides practical suggestions for everyday living with vision loss on topics such as lighting, home safety, leisure, communication, and labeling. LP, C, and B. $3.00

SOURCES OF AIDS AND DEVICES

Unless otherwise noted, the following vendors offer a range of products, including talking items, magnifiers, kitchen aids, recreational products, and computers. Catalogues are FREE and in standard print, unless otherwise noted.

ADAPTABILITY
PO Box 515
Colchester, CT 06415-0515
(800) 266-8856   FAX (800) 566-6678

ANN MORRIS ENTERPRISES
890 Fams Court
East Meadow, NY 11554
(800) 454-3175   (516) 292-9232

Catalogue available in LP, C, and PC disk; FREE. Braille catalogue, $10.00.

CORNING MEDICAL OPTICS
MP 21-2-2
Corning, NY 14831
(800) 742-5273   (607) 974-7823

Sells glare control lenses that filter out ultraviolet light and certain blue wavelengths. For people with photophobia.

FLORIDA NEW CONCEPTS MARKETING
PO Box 261
Port Richey, FL 34673
(800) 456-7097

Sells Beam Scope, which enlarges television picture up to two times. Prices vary with screen size.

INDEPENDENT LIVING AIDS, INC. (ILA)
27 East Mall
Plainview, NY 11803
(800) 537-2118   (516) 752-8080

Standard print catalogue. Also available in voice indexed cassette for $3.00, which may be applied to an order.

LIGHTHOUSE LOW VISION PRODUCTS
36-20 Northern Boulevard
Long Island City, NY 11101
(800) 453-4923   FAX (718) 786-0437

LP catalogue.

LS & S GROUP
PO Box 673
Northbrook, IL 60065
(800) 468-4789   (708) 498-9777

Catalogues in P (free) and C ($3.00, applied to purchase.)

MEDIC ALERT
PO Box 1009
Turlock, CA 95381-1009
(800) 344-3226   In CA, (209) 668-3333

Medical identification bracelet for people with chronic eye conditions and other diseases.

MONS INTERNATIONAL
PO Box 941621
Atlanta, GA 30341
(800) 541-7903   In Atlanta, (404) 551-8455

NATIONAL FEDERATION OF THE BLIND
Materials Center
1800 Johnson Street
Baltimore, MD 21230
(410) 659-9314

P, B, or PC disk; FREE.

SCIENCE PRODUCTS
Box 888
Southeastern, PA 19399
(800) 888-7400   FAX (215) 296-0488

"Vision Aids Resource Guide" offers optical and nonoptical aids. "Technilog" offers specially adapted scientific and technical instruments plus standard aids. "Magnilog" features magnifiers and adaptive aids for everyday living.

SEARS HOME HEALTHCARE CATALOG
Sears, Roebuck and Co.
20 Presidential Drive
Roselle, IL 60172
(800) 326-1750   (800) 733-7249 (TT)

Sells health care products. Sears Home HealthCare will file for Medicare reimbursement for customers. In-home or on-site service available.

VISUAL AIDS AND INFORMATIONAL MATERIAL
National Association for the Visually Handicapped (NAVH)
22 West 21st Street
New York, NY 10010
(212) 889-3141

LP catalogue.

RECREATION AND TRAVEL

Many individuals who have low vision need assistance in order to continue with their favorite hobbies or recreational pastimes. Others may develop an interest in a new hobby or sport as a means of socializing with organized groups or individuals.

Staff at the state agency that serves individuals who are visually impaired or blind can make referrals to organizations and groups that conduct special programs, including beep baseball, cross-country and downhill skiing, crafts courses, and other adult recreational programs.

Travel and recreation opportunities for people with vision loss have expanded greatly in recent years. In the U.S. and Canada, many state and provincial tourism offices provide information about accessible attractions for prospective visitors who are visually impaired or blind or have other disabilities. Auto clubs both here and abroad are also good sources of such information.

When planning trips, it is wise to contact hotels and tourist attractions in advance to ask about accessibility for people with vision loss. Some museums and historical sites have special tours, literature in LARGE PRINT, or tour guides on audiocassette. Hotel chains, airlines, and car rental companies provide special assistance to people with disabilities. Some companies offer specially trained travel companions to people with disabilities who need an escort. The growing number of travel agencies that plan trips for people with disabilities can provide assistance in obtaining this information.

Amtrak offers a 25% discount on a regular one-way coach fare for adults with disabilities and 50% for children ages 2 to 11. Passengers must present proof of disability, such as a certificate of legal blindness or a letter from a physician specifying the nature of the disability. Greyhound allows a passenger with a disability and a companion who will provide assistance in boarding/exiting the bus to travel for the price of a single adult fare. There is no charge for guide dogs for individuals who are visually impaired, blind, or deaf.

The Federal Aviation Administration requires each airline to submit a company-wide policy for travelers with disabilities. Passengers may call ahead to request early boarding, special seating, or meals which meet dietary restrictions.

Individuals who are legally blind are eligible for special entrance passes to federal recreation facilities. The Golden Access Passport is a FREE lifetime pass available to any U.S. citizen or permanent resident, regardless of age, who is legally blind or permanently disabled. It admits the permit holder and passengers in a single, private, noncommercial vehicle to any parks, monuments, historic sites, recreation areas, and wildlife refuges which usually charge entrance fees. If the permit holder does not enter by car, the Passport admits the permit holder, spouse, and children. The permit holder is also entitled to a 50% discount on charges such as camping, boat launching, and parking fees. Fees charged by private concessionaires are not discounted. Golden Access Passports are available only in person, with proof of disability, such as a certificate of legal blindness. Since the Passport is available at most federal recreation areas, it is not necessary to obtain one ahead of time.

Special camp programs are sponsored by organizations that serve people who are visually impaired or blind; other camp programs integrate sighted campers with people who are visually impaired or blind. In addition to traditional summer camp programs, some organizations offer week-long and weekend programs throughout the year. Financial aid is often available.

ORGANIZATIONS

NATIONAL CAMPS FOR THE BLIND
Christian Record Services
4444 South 52nd Street, Box 6097
Lincoln, NE 68506
(402) 488-0981   (402) 488-1902 (TT)
FAX (402) 488-7582

Sponsors more than 25 youth, youth/adult, and winter camps in the U.S. and Canada for individuals who are visually impaired, blind, hard-of-hearing, or deaf. FREE except for $25.00 processing fee.

NATIONAL LIBRARY SERVICE FOR THE BLIND AND PHYSICALLY HANDICAPPED (NLS)
1291 Taylor Street, NW
Washington, DC 20542
(800) 424-8567 or 8572 (Reference Section)
(202) 707-5100   FAX (202) 707-0712

Produces reference circulars, including "Sports, Outdoor Recreation, and Games for Visually and Physically Impaired Individuals," which lists national organizations, literature, and sources for adapted sports equipment and games, and "Leisure Pursuit Bibliographies," which list books available through the NLS. Subjects include birding, fishing, sailing, and swimming. Bibliographies are available in LP, disc, and B; FREE.

NATIONAL PARK SERVICE
Department of the Interior, Office of Public Affairs
PO Box 37127
Washington, DC 20013-7127
(202) 208-4747

Operates the Golden Access Passport program for people who are legally blind or have other disabilities. FREE brochure.

TRAVELIN' TALK
PO Box 3534
Clarksville, TN 37043-3534
(615) 552-6670

A network of individuals and organizations that provides assistance to travelers with disabilities. One time registration fee varies according to income. Newsletter, "Travelin' Talk," P, LP, and C; annual contribution for newsletter requested.

VERY SPECIAL ARTS
John F. Kennedy Center for the Performing Arts
Washington, DC 20566
(202) 628-2800   (202) 737-0645 (TT)
FAX (202) 737-0725

Provides opportunities for individuals with disabilities to participate in fine and performing arts.

PUBLICATIONS AND TAPES

CC INC. AUTO TAPE TOURS
PO Box 227/2 Elbrook Drive
Allendale, NJ 07401
(201) 236-1666

Audiocassettes and videotapes that serve as previews for trips or walking tour guides. FREE catalogue.

CRAFTS RESOURCES IN SPECIAL MEDIA
VISION Foundation, Inc.
818 Mt. Auburn Street
Watertown, MA 02172
(617) 926-4232   In MA, (800) 852-3029
FAX (617) 926-1412

A LARGE PRINT list of instruction manuals, kits, and other resources available in LP, C, and B; FREE.

EASY ACCESS TO NATIONAL PARKS: THE SIERRA CLUB GUIDE FOR PEOPLE WITH DISABILITIES
by Wendy Roth and Michael Tompane
Sierra Club Books
100 Bush Street, 13 Floor
San Francisco, CA 94104
(800) 733-3000

Reviews accessibility of 50 national parks for individuals with vision, hearing, or mobility impairments. $16.00 plus $4.00 shipping and handling. Available in braille from the

National Library Service for the Blind and Physically Handicapped, 1291 Taylor Street, NW, Washington, DC 20542.

FODOR'S GREAT AMERICAN VACATIONS FOR TRAVELERS WITH DISABILITIES
201 East 50th Street
New York, NY 10022
(800) 733-3000

Includes accessibility information for hotels, restaurants and attractions. U.S., $18.00; Canada, $24.00; plus $4.00 shipping and handling.

GUIDE TO ACCREDITED CAMPS
American Camping Association (ACA)
5000 State Road 67 North
Martinsville, IN 46151
(800) 428-2267   (317) 342-8456
FAX (317) 342-2065

This guide of ACA-accredited camps includes special programs for campers with disabilities. $10.95

GUIDE TO SUMMER CAMPS AND SUMMER SCHOOLS
Porter Sargent Publishers, Inc.
11 Beacon Street, Suite 1400
Boston, MA 02108
(617) 523-1670   FAX (617) 523-1021

This guide to summer educational and recreation programs includes special programs for individuals with disabilities. $25.00 plus $2.74 shipping and handling.

GUILD FOR THE BLIND
180 North Michigan Avenue
Chicago, IL 60601
(312) 236-8569

Publishes instruction books for crafts such as needlework, macrame, and sewing and cookbooks in LP, C, and B. FREE catalogue.

HORIZONS FOR THE BLIND
16A Meadowdale Shopping Center
Carpentersville, IL 60110-2075
(708) 836-1400   In IL, (800) 318-2000
FAX (708) 826-1443

Publishes crafts instruction manuals in LP and B. Quarterly newsletter, "On the Horizon," LP and B; FREE.

LARGE PRINT PUBLISHING COMPANY
103 Forest Glen
West Springfield, MA 01089
(413) 739-0894

Publishes LP puzzles, including crosswords, trivia, and circle word puzzles, and adult coloring designs. FREE sample pack; $5.50, shipping and handling.

POPULAR ACTIVITIES & GAMES FOR BLIND, VISUALLY IMPAIRED, & DISABLED PEOPLE

American Foundation for the Blind (AFB)
c/o American Book Center
Brooklyn Navy Yard, Building No. 3
Brooklyn, NY 11205
(718) 852-9873   FAX (718) 935-9647

Lists 50 indoor and outdoor games and activities suitable for individuals of all ages. LP. $16.95 plus $3.50 shipping

WORLDWIDE GAMES

PO Box 517
Colchester, CT 06415-0517
(800) 243-9232   FAX (800) 566-6678

Catalogue of games and crafts.

Chapter 8

SERVICES FOR ELDERS

Visual impairment is one of the most common impairments among the population age 65 years or older. A recent study reported that 16 percent of Americans in this age category had difficulty reading letters and words in ordinary newsprint even when wearing corrective lenses; of this total 3.3 percent could not see letters or words at all (McNeil:1993).

There are numerous eye conditions related to aging, but the four leading causes of vision loss in elders are macular degeneration, cataracts, glaucoma, and diabetic eye disease. (See Chapter 12, "SPECIAL SERVICES AND PRODUCTS BY EYE DISEASE/CONDITION.")

Many elders accept vision loss and other disabilities as a "normal part of aging" and therefore do not seek out services. A recent study found that elders residing in nursing homes experienced blindness at rates higher than their counterparts living in the community (13 times higher for African Americans and nearly 16 times higher for whites). The authors suggested that over 40 percent of the blindness could be prevented or treated, most notably through cataract extraction (Tielsch et al.: 1995).

With the help of rehabilitation services and assistive devices, elders are able to adapt to vision loss as success-fully as other age groups. When other disabling condi-tions are present, elders must be certain to inform service

LIVING WITH LOW VISION: A Resource Guide for People with Sight Loss, Lexington, MA: Resources for Rehabilitation, Copyright 1996

providers so that additional accommodations may be made. For example, an elder who has a tremor may find it difficult to use a hand held magnifier for reading but may work effectively with a stand magnifier.

Vision loss often has an effect on other health conditions. For example, elders, especially those with osteoporosis, are susceptible to fractures of the hip and other bones when they fall; vision loss is often the cause of falls among elders. The inability to drive may prevent elders from seeking out proper medical care for other health conditions. Many times agencies that serve individuals who are visually impaired or blind and agencies that serve elders arrange for transportation to medical appointments for their clients.

The combination of vision loss and hearing loss, which is common among elders, may have a great effect on the ability to function. Individuals with hearing loss use visual cues to help them understand conversations; vision loss decreases the ability to do this and may result in a feeling of extreme isolation. Special services for individuals with dual sensory losses are available at both public and private agencies.

Elders may need services from a rehabilitation teacher or occupational therapist in order to continue carrying out the activities of everyday living. Obtaining appropriate rehabilitation services can prevent unnecessary placement in nursing homes and other long-term care facilities.

Elders living with family members may be fearful of losing their independence if their spouse or another family member becomes overly protective and tries to do everything for them. In such instances, it is often useful to seek out family counseling or to attend a self-help group that includes family members.

Both public and private organizations as well as self-help groups are available to assist elders with vision loss in most major metropolitan areas. The state agency that serves individuals who are visually impaired or blind is also a good source of information and may provide special services to elders with vision loss, often as part of a federally funded program of Independent Living Services for Older Blind Individuals.

Senior centers, home health care providers, geriatric case managers, and special services for elders located at hospitals should all be able to accommodate the special needs of elders with vision loss and other disabilities. Often senior centers provide vision screenings and special transportation services that can be invaluable to elders with vision loss. In some communities, public libraries have special programs for elders or for patrons who are unable to get to the library.

References

McNeil, John M.
1993 AMERICANS WITH DISABILITIES 1991-1992, Washington, DC: U.S. Bureau of the Census Current Population Reports P70-33

Tielsch, James M., Jonathan C. Javitt, Anne Coleman, Joanne Katz, and Alfred Sommer
1995 "The Prevalence of Blindness and Visual Impairment

Among Nursing Home Residents in Baltimore" NEW ENGLAND JOURNAL OF MEDICINE 332:18(May 4):1205-1209

ORGANIZATIONS

ELDERCARE LOCATOR
National Association of Area Agencies on Aging (NAAAA)
(800) 677-1116   (202) 296-8130

A nationwide information and referral service that provides callers with the phone number for an information and referral service, which in turn provides the name of a local agency that addresses the caller's specific needs. FREE.

LIGHTHOUSE NATIONAL CENTER FOR VISION AND AGING (NCVA)
111 East 59th Street
New York, NY 10022
(800) 334-5497 (V/TT)   (212) 821-9200
(212) 821-9713 (TT)   FAX (212) 821-9705

Provides information on vision problems faced by older people and how these problems can be treated. Sells community education materials. FREE newsletter.

NATIONAL INSTITUTE ON AGING (NIA)
NIA Information Center
PO Box 8057
Gaithersburg, MD 20898-8057
(301) 495-3455

Clearinghouse for information on aging. Publishes LP fact sheet series, "Age Page," which focuses on issues faced by elders, including "Aging and Your Eyes," FREE.

AGING AND VISION LOSS

Resources for Rehabilitation
33 Bedford Street, Suite 19A
Lexington, MA 02173
(617) 862-6455   FAX (617) 861-7517

A LARGE PRINT (18 point bold type) publication that describes organizations and publications for elders with vision loss. Minimum purchase, 25 copies. $1.25 per copy plus shipping and handling. Discounts available for purchases of 100 or more copies. See order form on last page of this book.

CARING FOR THE VISUALLY IMPAIRED OLDER PERSON

Vision Loss Resources
1936 Lyndale Avenue South
Minneapolis, MN 55403
(612) 871-2222 (V/TT, FAX)

Intended as a guide for long-term care facility staff, this booklet offers many helpful suggestions for anyone facing vision loss. $10.00 plus $2.50 shipping and handling.

COPING WITH THE DIAGNOSIS OF SIGHT LOSS

Resources for Rehabilitation
33 Bedford Street, Suite 19A
Lexington, MA 02173
(617) 862-6455   FAX (617) 861-7517

An audiocassette in which three consumers, two of them over age 55, discuss their experiences after they became visually impaired. $12.00 plus $3.00 shipping and handling.

EIGHTY-EIGHT EASY-TO-MAKE AIDS FOR OLDER PEOPLE
by Don Caston
Hartley & Marks Publishers
Box 147
Point Roberts, WA 98281
(206) 945-2017

Practical adaptations for the home with step-by-step instructions. $11.95 plus $1.50 postage and handling.

A HANDBOOK FOR SENIOR CITIZENS: RIGHTS, RESOURCES AND RESPONSIBILITIES
by Ramona Walhof
National Federation of the Blind (NFB)
1800 Johnson Street
Baltimore, MD 21230
(410) 659-9314   FAX (410) 685-5653

Practical advice for individuals with vision loss, their families, and professionals working with them. P, $7.00; C, FREE.

I KEEP FIVE PAIRS OF GLASSES IN A FLOWER POT
by Henrietta Levner
National Association for Visually Handicapped (NAVH)
22 West 21st Street
New York, NY 10010
(212) 889-3141

Describes an older woman's experience in learning to live with low vision caused by macular degeneration. LP. Members, $2.00; nonmembers, $3.00.

LIVING WITH VISION LOSS: A HANDBOOK FOR CARE-GIVERS
Canadian National Institute for the Blind (CNIB)
Rehabilitation Department
1929 Bayview Avenue
Toronto, Ontario M4G 3E8 Canada
(416) 480-7626   FAX (416) 480-7677

Practical suggestions for everyday living with visual impairment or blindness. Includes community and CNIB resources. $12.50, Canadian funds

OUT OF THE CORNER OF MY EYE: LIVING WITH VISION LOSS IN LATER LIFE
by Nicolette Pernod Ringgold
American Foundation for the Blind (AFB)
c/o American Book Center
Brooklyn Navy Yard, Building No. 3
Brooklyn, NY 11205
(718) 852-9873   FAX (718) 935-9647

Written by a woman who became legally blind due to macular degeneration in her late 70's, this book offers practical advice and encouragement for elders with vision loss. LP and C, $19.95 plus $3.50 shipping and handling.

RESOURCES FOR ELDERS WITH DISABILITIES
Resources for Rehabilitation
33 Bedford Street, Suite 19A
Lexington, MA 02173
(617) 862-6455   FAX (617) 861-7517

A LARGE PRINT resource directory that describes services and products that elders with disabilities need to function independently. Includes chapters on vision loss, hearing loss, arthritis, diabetes, osteoporosis, Parkinson's disease, falls, and stroke. $43.95 plus $5.00 shipping and handling. See order form on last page of this book.

SEE FOR YOURSELF
The Lighthouse, Inc.
111 East 59th Street
New York, NY 10022
(800) 334-5497 (V/TT)   (212) 821-9200
(212) 821-9713 (TT)   FAX (212) 821-9705

This videotape portrays elders with vision loss living independently using low vision aids and other assistive devices. Close-captioned. $50.00. Available in English and Spanish.

TALKING BOOKS FOR SENIOR ADULTS
National Library Service for the Blind and Physically Handicapped (NLS)
1291 Taylor Street NW
Washington, DC 20542
(800) 424-8567 or 8572 (Reference Section)
(202) 707-5100   FAX (202) 707-0712

This brochure promotes the use of talking books by seniors and describes how to receive them. Available in English and Spanish. FREE.

THROUGH GRANDPA'S EYES
by Patricia MacLachlan
Harper Collins
PO Box 588
Dunmore, PA 18512
(800) 331-3761

In this children's story, a young boy learns how his grandfather sees by using his senses of hearing, touch, and smell. $14.89 plus $2.75 shipping and handling. Also available on audiocassette on loan from the National Library Service for the Blind and Physically Handicapped regional libraries, RC 25436.

THE WORLD THROUGH THEIR EYES

The Lighthouse, Inc.
111 East 59th Street
New York, NY 10022
(800) 334-5497 (V/TT)   (212) 821-9200
(212) 821-9713 (TT)   FAX (212) 821-9705

This videotape portrays elders with vision loss living in a long term care facility and shows how staff can enhance residents' independence through the use of assistive devices such as low vision aids. Accompanying manual discusses common types of visual impairment. $25.00

Chapter 9

SERVICES FOR CHILDREN AND ADOLESCENTS

It is not uncommon for children who experience vision loss to be premature infants who also experience a number of concurrent disabilities. Retinopathy of prematurity (ROP), a major cause of vision loss in children, involves the growth of abnormal blood vessels and scar tissue in the vitreous (the transparent gel that fills the eyeball) and retinal detachments; it is a condition that occurs in low birth weight premature babies. First observed in the 1940's, this condition was originally called retrolental fibroplasia (RLF) and attributed to the use of excessive oxygen in incubators; this single cause is no longer accepted. Most researchers agree that prematurity itself and low birth weight are primary contributors to retinopathy of prematurity.

Cryotherapy, which freezes peripheral areas of the retina in order to slow or reverse the development of abnormal blood vessels and scar tissue, is effective in a large number of cases that have reached a threshold level of the disease. Some investigators have found that Vitamin E is effective in the prevention of retinopathy of prematurity.

In order to obtain optimal treatment, parents should ensure that their premature babies receive regular ophthalmic examinations. Because children with retinopathy of prematurity are at risk for developing other eye conditions,

LIVING WITH LOW VISION: A Resource Guide for People with Sight Loss, Lexington, MA: Resources for Rehabilitation, Copyright 1996

these examinations should not cease after a few years, and teachers should be informed of the child's condition in order to report any unusual visual behavior.

EDUCATIONAL SERVICES

An appropriate public education for children with disabilities, including special education and related services, was mandated by the Education of the Handicapped Act (P.L. 94-142) passed in 1975. In 1990, the name of the Education of the Handicapped Act was changed to the Individuals with Disabilities Education Act, referred to as IDEA (P.L. 101-476). At the time this book went to press, Congress was debating the reauthorization of IDEA.

The law requires that an Individualized Education Plan (IEP) be developed for each student with special needs. The special education or vision teacher and parents work together to develop an IEP, which specifies educational goals, courses of instruction, special equipment, and other services to be provided. The vision teacher serves as the "case manager" and recommends the services of other team members such as orientation and mobility instructors. Parents have the right to appeal if they disagree with the school's decision and may arrange for an independent evaluation of their child.

Schools that serve large numbers of children who are visually impaired or blind employ full-time vision teachers. Schools with few students who are visually impaired or blind employ itinerant vision teachers, who often work for a collaborative of area schools. In public schools, children may receive instruction in subjects such as typing or braille in a specially equipped resource room or on an as-needed basis through consultation with the regular classroom teacher. Many of the special computer devices described in Chapter 6, "HIGH TECH AIDS," are appropriate for children to use in the classroom.

Many children with multiple disabilities including visual impairments are served by public school programs. However, some of these students may require a concentrated program that results in placement in a residential facility. Residential facilities may also offer a combination of educational resources needed by the gifted youngster who is visually impaired or blind, or these services may be available in programs for gifted students in public schools.

To obtain information about educational services, contact the local school system or the state department of special education. Special instruction for infants and toddlers with disabilities is available through federally funded programs. Call the local children's hospital or children's services agency in your area to ask about these early intervention programs.

Adolescents who are visually impaired or blind have special needs as they consider career goals and higher education. A separate section below lists funding sources for students with vision loss; student support groups and a special magazine for teens are also included.

OTHER SERVICES AND BENEFITS

State commissions that serve individuals who are visually impaired or blind may also offer services such as home visits, infant-toddler programs, counseling for parents, information and referral, funding for summer camp, after-school programs, and other supplementary services. (See "Appendix A: Main Offices of State Agencies that Serve Individuals Who are Visually Impaired or Blind"). In some states, children who are visually impaired or blind are not served by the state agency that serves adults. Contact the state department of special education for information. Services for children and adolescents with vision loss are also available at many local and national organizations. Many agencies also provide services to family members.

Some children with disabilities are eligible for monthly Social Security benefits if their family meets a financial means test. A recent court case found that Social Security's eligibility criteria for children during the 1980's did not reflect the intent of Congress, and as a result, disability evaluations for children have been changed. Children who were denied benefits from 1980 to 1990 may now be eligible and may also receive retroactive benefits. Contact the Social Security Administration [(800) 772-1213 or (800) 325-0778 (TT)] to determine whether your child is eligible for medical or cash benefits.

Because parents experience such intense emotional reactions to a child's visual impairment or blindness, counseling to help them cope with their own emotions will contribute to their ability to help the child. Such counseling may be available from medical professionals, social workers or psychologists, rehabilitation counselors, and other parents in similar situations. Talking with other parents either in private or at a parent support group helps parents to learn that their emotional responses are normal.

When there are other children in the family, there is a need to preserve a sense of normalcy and at the same time help the child who is visually impaired or blind. Siblings may be jealous of the attention that is paid to the child who is visually impaired or blind. Local agencies may provide help and support for parents and other family members. Some offer parent support groups, where members learn from each others' experiences about how to cope emotionally as well as how to find the resources to help their children develop.

ORGANIZATIONS

BEACH CENTER ON FAMILIES AND DISABILITY
c/o Institute for Life Span Studies
3111 Haworth Hall
Lawrence, KS 66045
(913) 864-7600 (V/TT)   FAX (913) 864-7605

A federally funded center that conducts research and training related to families with members who have disabilities. Publications catalogue describes monographs and tapes related to family coping, professional roles, and service delivery; FREE. Publishes newsletter, "Families and Disability," FREE.

CANADIAN NATIONAL INSTITUTE FOR THE BLIND (CNIB)
1929 Bayview Avenue
Toronto, Ontario M4G 3E8 Canada
(416) 480-7580   FAX (416) 480-7677

Provides counseling, life skills training, sight enhancement services, summer youth programs, teen and parent support groups, library services, and career development programs. Services vary from office to office (See "Appendix B: Division Offices of the Canadian National Institute for the Blind").

CLEARINGHOUSE ON DISABILITY INFORMATION
Office of Special Education and Rehabilitative Services (OSERS)
U.S. Department of Education
Room 3132 Switzer Building
Washington, DC 20202-2524
(202) 205-8241 (V/TT)   (202) 205-8723 (V/TT)

Answers questions about services and programs for individuals of all ages with disabilities. Produces a variety of publications including newsletter, "OSERS in Print," which focuses on federal activities; FREE.

COUNCIL OF FAMILIES WITH VISUAL IMPAIRMENTS (CFVI)
American Council of the Blind
1155 15th Street NW, Suite 720
Washington, DC 20005
(800) 424-8666   (202) 467-5081
FAX (202) 467-5085

Consumer group for blind/sighted parents of blind/sighted children. Publishes newsletter, "Reflections," in LP and C.

GTE EDUCATIONAL NETWORK SERVICES
5525 MacArthur Boulevard, Suite 320
Irving, TX 75038
(800) 927-3000   FAX (214) 751-0964

Operates a wide number of databases and bulletin board

services for both parents of children with disabilities and professional service providers. Special topic bulletin boards include vision and deaf-blindness. Accessible by direct dial-up and through the Internet. One-time set-up fee, $25.00; annual fee, $35.00; minimum monthly usage charge, $14.00; online charges vary.

HADLEY SCHOOL FOR THE BLIND
700 Elm Street
Winnetka, IL 60093
(800) 323-4238   In IL, (708) 446-8111

Offers correspondence courses for parents of children who are visually impaired or blind; FREE. Course catalogue available in LP, C, and B; FREE.

HEATH RESOURCE CENTER
One Dupont Circle, Suite 800
Washington, DC 20036-1193
(800) 544-3284 (V/TT)   (202) 939-9320 (V/TT)
FAX (202) 833-4760

Provides information about the transition from high school to postsecondary education. Publishes newsletter, "Information from HEATH," three times a year. Publishes "Students Who are Blind or Visually Impaired in Postsecondary Education," "Career Planning and Employment Strategies," "How to Choose a College: Guide for the Student with a Disability" and "Vocational Rehabilitation Services: A Postsecondary Student Consumer's Guide." Publications list and all HEATH publications are FREE in P,

C, and disk (DOS or Mac).

KIDS ON THE BLOCK
9385-C Gerwig Lane
Columbia, MD 21046
(800) 368-5437   (410) 290-9095
FAX (410) 290-9358

A program that uses puppets to help students understand disabilities and chronic conditions. Various programs available, including blindness, diabetes, and sibling of a disabled child. Also publishes "The Kids on the Block" series of books, written for children in grades two to five, which feature children with chronic conditions or disabilities. "Business is Looking Up" is the story of a youngster with visual impairment who starts a small business. Question and answer sections about the characters' disabilities in each book. $12.95

LEARNING PILLOWS
PO Box 345
Greenfield, NH 03047-0345
(603) 547-2446

Puppets and pillows, including Mr. Bug, Bumpedy Bumps, and the King and His Closet, that help young children with eye-hand coordination, visual discrimination, buttoning, and zipping, etc. Some pillows have coordinated stories on audiocassette and a parent/teacher activity guide. Prices range from $8.00 for puppets to $30.00 for pillows and audiocassettes plus shipping and handling.

LIGHTHOUSE NATIONAL CENTER FOR VISION AND CHILD DEVELOPMENT (NCVCD)
111 East 59th Street
New York, NY 10022
(800) 334-5497 (V/TT)   (212) 821-9200
(212) 821-9713 (TT)   FAX (212) 821-9705

Promotes understanding of vision loss in children and adolescents, child development, special education, and parent-teacher-professional cooperation. Publishes newsletter, "EnVision," three times/year; FREE.

LINCS-BBS
Family Resource Center for Children with Special Needs
535 Race Street, #140
San Jose, CA 95126
BBS (408) 294-6933   FAX (408) 288-7943

Provides information to parents of children with special needs and service providers. No online or registration fees. Individuals who do not have a computer should contact the LINCS Project Coordinator for more information.

NATIONAL ALLIANCE OF BLIND STUDENTS
c/o American Council of the Blind (ACB)
1155 15th Street, NW, Suite 720
Washington, DC 20005
(800) 424-8666   (202) 467-5081
FAX (202) 467-5085

Consumer group for college students who are visually impaired or blind. Publishes "The Student Advocate," three times per year, in LP and C. Membership, $5.00.

NATIONAL ASSOCIATION FOR PARENTS OF VISUALLY IMPAIRED (NAPVI)
PO Box 317
Watertown, MA 02272-0317
(800) 562-6265   FAX (617) 972-7444

Promotes development of parent groups; provides information through conferences, publications, and quarterly newsletter, "Awareness." Local chapters in some states. FREE information packet. Membership, $20.00.

NATIONAL ASSOCIATION FOR VISUALLY HANDICAPPED (NAVH)
22 West 21st Street
New York, NY 10010
(212) 889-3141

Sells and lends LP books for children. LP newsletter for youth, "In Focus," FREE.

NATIONAL CENTER FOR YOUTH WITH DISABILITIES (NCYD)
University of Minnesota
Box 721 UMHC
Harvard Street at East River Road
Minneapolis, MN 55455
(800) 333-6293   (612) 626-2825
(612) 624-3939 (TT)   FAX (612) 626-2134

An information center on adolescents with chronic illness and disabilities that provides access to research findings, resources, and advocacy for professional service providers and for parents. Maintains a national resource database and library with abstracts of current literature on disability and chronic illness; information about innovative programs; and a network of consultants who provide technical assistance. Publishes newsletter, "Connections," FREE.

NATIONAL FEDERATION OF THE BLIND (NFB)
1800 Johnson Street
Baltimore, MD 21230
(410) 659-9314   FAX (410) 685-5653

The Parents of Blind Children Division sponsors seminars and workshops and provides information and support. Publishes "Future Reflections," a quarterly magazine with resources and guidelines, P and C. Membership, $8.00. FREE Parents Information Pack. Also produces two books on education of blind children: "Your School Includes a Blind Student," $3.75, and "A Resource Guide for Parents and Educators of Blind Children," $5.95. NFB's Student

Division provides support to students through chapters in many states.

NATIONAL INFORMATION CENTER FOR CHILDREN AND YOUTH WITH DISABILITIES (NICHCY)
PO Box 1492
Washington, DC 20013-1492
(800) 695-0285 (V/TT)   (202) 884-8200 (V/TT)
FAX (202) 884-8441

A federally funded clearinghouse that provides information about disabilities and referral guides. Publishes newsletter, "News Digest," which focuses on special topics such as "Assistive Technology," "Children with Handicaps, Parent and Family Issues," and "Understanding Sibling Issues," FREE.

NATIONAL LIBRARY SERVICE FOR THE BLIND AND PHYSICALLY HANDICAPPED (NLS)
1291 Taylor Street NW
Washington, DC 20542
(800) 424-8567 or 8572 (Reference Section)
(202) 707-5100   FAX (202) 707-0712

Provides talking book equipment and recorded and braille books for preschoolers, students, and adults through a network of regional libraries. Publishes "Parents' Guide to the Development of Pre-School Handicapped Children: Resources and Services," "Selected Readings for Parents of Preschool Handicapped Children," and "From School to Working Life: Resources and Services," FREE.

PACER CENTER (PARENT ADVOCACY COALITION FOR EDUCATIONAL RIGHTS)

4826 Chicago Avenue South
Minneapolis, MN 55417-1098
(612) 827-2966 (V/TT)   In MN, (800) 537-2237
FAX (612) 827-3065

A coalition of disability organizations which offers information about laws, procedures, and parents' rights and responsibilities. Publishes the "Pacesetter," three times per year, FREE; the "Advocate," six times per year, $15.00; "Early Childhood Connection," for parents of young children with disabilities, three times per year, FREE. Materials are available in LP, C, and B upon request. Edits two bulletin boards on GTE Educational Network Services, PIP (Programs Involving Parents) and ADA.INDEPENDENT. (See GTE EDUCATIONAL NETWORK SERVICES listing below). FREE catalogue.

PARENT EDUCATION AND ASSISTANCE FOR KIDS (PEAK)

6055 Lehman Drive, Suite 101
Colorado Springs, CO 80918
(800) 284-0251   (719) 531-9400
(719) 531-9403 (V/TT)   FAX (719) 531-9452

A center that promotes the integration of children with disabilities in the regular classroom. Provides referrals for parents and technical assistance to school systems. Publishes newsletter, "Speak Out" (in English and Spanish), $9.00 for out of state professionals; FREE for others.

PUBLICATIONS AND TAPES

AMERICAN PRINTING HOUSE FOR THE BLIND (APH)
1839 Frankfort Avenue
Louisville, KY 40206-0085
(800) 223-1839   (502) 895-2405
FAX (502) 895-1509

Sells infant, preschool, kindergarten, primary, and multi-handicapped aids including games, teaching aids, and texts. Titles include "Beginnings--A Practical Guide for Parents and Teachers of Visually Impaired Babies," $7.50; "Hands On: Functional Activities for Visually Impaired Preschoolers," "Parents and Visually Impaired Infants," $26.00, and a videotape, "Playing the Crucial Role in Your Child's Development," $20.75. Request a preschool packet. Also publishes "Century Series Braille Books," fiction and nonfiction titles sold at the same prices as standard print books.

BLIND CHILDRENS CENTER
4120 Marathon Street
PO Box 29159
Los Angeles, CA 90029-0159
(800) 222-3566   In CA, (800) 222-3567
(213) 664-2153   FAX (213) 665-3828

Provides resources and support to parents. Publications include "First Steps: A Handbook for Teaching Young Children Who Are Visually Impaired," $28.00; "Talk to Me I," "Talk to Me II," "Heart-to-Heart - Parents of Blind and

Partially Sighted Children Talk About Their Feelings,"
"Move with Me," and "Learning to Play: Common Concerns for the Visually Impaired Preschool Child," $2.00
each; "Dancing Cheek to Cheek," $4.00; and "Reaching,
Crawling, Walking: Let's Get Moving," $4.00.

BOOMERANG!
13366 Pescadero Road
La Honda, CA 94020
(800) 333-7858

Monthly current events magazine for children on standard
audiocassette. $39.95 for 12 issues; $7.95 for a single
issue.

BUILDING INTEGRATION WITH THE I.E.P.
by Barbara E. Buswell and Judy Veneris
Parent Education and Assistance for Kids (PEAK)
6055 Lehman Drive, Suite 101
Colorado Springs, CO 80918
(800) 284-0251   (719) 531-9400
(719) 531-9403 (V/TT)   FAX (719) 531-9452

A booklet that helps parents understand what they can do
and expect from the I.E.P. meetings. $5.00

CAN DO VIDEO SERIES
Visually Impaired Preschool Services
1229 Garvin Place
Louisville, KY 40203
(502) 636-3207   FAX (502) 636-0024

A series of five videotapes that depict six families with children who are visually impaired, ranging from 14 months to six years. Write for description of tapes. Each tape may be purchased separately for $39.95 or the entire set may be purchased for $179.95. $10.00 shipping charge for up to five tapes.

CHILDREN'S BRAILLE BOOK CLUB
National Braille Press (NBP)
88 St. Stephen Street
Boston, MA 02115
(617) 266-6160   FAX (617) 437-0456

Braille pages are inserted into standard print children's books. FREE membership provides monthly notices with no obligation to buy; $100.00 annual subscription automatically provides one print-braille book per month.

CORNERSTONE BOOKS
801 94th Avenue North
St. Petersburg, FL 33702
(800) 879-4459   FAX (800) 473-7090

LP fiction for children and adolescents. FREE catalogue.

DIRECTORY OF COLLEGE FACILITIES AND SERVICES FOR PEOPLE WITH DISABILITIES
Oryx Press, Phoenix, AZ
(800) 279-6799   FAX (800) 279-4663

Describes the physical facilities, special services, and

academic programs for colleges throughout the U.S. and Canada. $115.00

THE EXCEPTIONAL PARENT
PO Box 3000, Dept. EP
Denville, NJ 07834
(800) 247-8080

This magazine emphasizes problem solving and provides practical information about raising and educating a child with a disability. Individuals, $24.00; schools, libraries, and agencies, $30.00.

GETTING IN TOUCH WITH PLAY: CREATIVE PLAY ENVIRONMENTS FOR CHILDREN WITH VISUAL IMPAIRMENTS
The Lighthouse, Inc.
111 East 59th Street
New York, NY 10022
(800) 334-5497 (V/TT)   (212) 821-9200
(212) 821-9713 (TT)   FAX (212) 821-9705

A book that includes a set of diagrams and photographs of playground settings that encourage children with visual impairments to play. $8.00

GUIDE TO RESOURCES FOR CHILDREN AND YOUTH WITH VISUAL IMPAIRMENTS
by Denise Ferrin
PO Box 11
Westminster, CA 92684

Lists organizations, services, and products. Includes section on computer products and services. $15.00 plus $2.00 shipping and handling.

GUIDE TO TOYS FOR CHILDREN WHO ARE BLIND OR VISUALLY IMPAIRED
American Toy Institute, Inc.
200 Fifth Avenue, Suite 740
New York, NY 10010
(800) 851-9955   (212) 675-1141
FAX (212) 633-1429

This booklet recommends toys appropriate for children with visual impairments, including toys for infants and preschoolers, dolls and stuffed toys, balls, games, building and musical toys, and vehicles; FREE.

INDIVIDUALIZED EDUCATION PROGRAMS (Reprint 2/90)
National Information Center for Children and Youth with Disabilities (NICHCY)
PO Box 1492
Washington, DC 20013
(800) 695-0285 (V/TT)   (202) 884-8200 (V/TT)
FAX (202) 884-8441

This publication describes the purposes and contents of the IEP, the responsibility of the state education agency, the role of parents, and the requirements for holding meetings. FREE.

JUST ENOUGH TO KNOW BETTER
by Eileen Curran
National Braille Press (NBP)
88 St. Stephen Street
Boston, MA 02115
(617) 266-6160   FAX (617) 437-0456

This self-paced workbook teaches beginning braille skills to sighted parents. $15.00

LIFEPRINTS
Blindskills, Inc.
Box 5181
Salem, OR 97304
(503) 581-4224   FAX (503) 581-1078

Magazine with focus on careers and life skills of youth and adults who are visually impaired or blind. LP, C, and B subscriptions, $20.00. Sample copy, $6.00.

LOW VISION: A RESOURCE GUIDE WITH ADAPTATIONS FOR STUDENTS WITH VISUAL IMPAIRMENTS
by Nancy Levack
Texas School for the Blind and Visually Impaired
Business Office
1100 West 45th Street
Austin, TX 78756-3494
(512) 454-8631   FAX (512) 458-3395

Provides functional vision assessment guidelines, medical information about eye diseases and conditions, and strategies for adapting materials and classroom environment for students with visual impairments. $20.00

OPENING DOORS: STRATEGIES FOR INCLUDING ALL STUDENTS IN REGULAR EDUCATION
by C. Beth Schaffner and Barbara E. Buswell
Parent Education and Assistance for Kids (PEAK)
6055 Lehman Drive, Suite 101
Colorado Springs, CO 80918
(800) 284-0251   (719) 531-9400
(719) 531-9403 (V/TT)   FAX (719) 531-9452

Written for educators and parents, this book contains practical information about integrating students with disabilities into regular classrooms. $10.00

QUESTIONS KIDS ASK ABOUT BLINDNESS
National Federation of the Blind (NFB)
1800 Johnson Street
Baltimore, MD 21230
(410) 659-9314   FAX (410) 685-5653

Answers general questions about blindness, braille, canes, guide dogs, and the abilities of individuals who are visually impaired or blind. Describes a typical day in the life of a blind sixth grader attending public school. $5.00

SEEDLINGS
PO Box 2395
Livonia, MI 48151-0395
(800) 777-8552   (313) 427-8552

Publishes inexpensive children's storybooks in braille. FREE catalogue.

SINCE OWEN
by Charles R. Callanan
Johns Hopkins University Press
2715 North Charles Street
Baltimore, MD 21218-4319
(800) 537-5487

Written by the father of a child with a disability, this book describes the experience of obtaining an appropriate education and finding resources. $16.95

THE STUDENT WITH ALBINISM IN THE REGULAR CLASS-ROOM
by Julia Robertson Ashley
National Organization for Albinism and Hypopigmentation (NOAH)
1530 Locust Street, #29
Philadelphia, PA 19102
(800) 473-2310   (215) 545-2322

Describes special needs of children with albinism and suggests adaptations for classroom and nonclassroom activities. LP, $4.00.

THEY DON'T COME WITH MANUALS
Fanlight Productions
47 Halifax Street
Boston, MA 02130
(800) 937-4113   (617) 524-0980
FAX (617) 524-8838

A videotape in which parents talk about their own experiences raising a child with a disability. 29 minutes Rental: $50.00 a day; $100.00 a week. Purchase: $195.00.

TRAVEL TALES - A MOBILITY STORYBOOK
Mostly Mobility
7100 Route 183
Bethel, PA 19507
(717) 933-5681

Designed to teach mobility to children in preschool through third grade, this book may be used by parents, classroom teachers, special education teachers, and orientation and mobility teachers. $22.00

TROLL LARGE PRINT
100 Corporate Drive
Mahwah, NJ 07430
(800) 929-8265   FAX (800) 979-8765

Modern classics for children, grades K to 9. $15.95 each. FREE catalogue.

FUNDING SOURCES FOR STUDENTS WITH VISION LOSS

Financial aid for students with disabilities is provided by the U.S. Department of Education and administered by state departments of vocational rehabilitation. Each state has its own eligibility criteria. Contact your state agency for more information (See "Appendix A: Main Offices of State Agencies that Serve Individuals Who are Visually Impaired or Blind").

The following organizations offer academic scholarships. Special qualification criteria are noted when applicable.

ORGANIZATIONS

AMERICAN COUNCIL OF THE BLIND (ACB)
Attn: Stephanie Cooper
1155 15th Street NW, Suite 720
Washington, DC 20005
(800) 424-8666   (202) 467-5081
FAX (202) 467-5085

AMERICAN FOUNDATION FOR THE BLIND (AFB)
11 Penn Plaza, Suite 300
New York, NY 10001
(212) 502-7600   FAX (212) 502-7774
Information line (800) 232-5463
In New York state, (212) 502-7657

ASSOCIATION FOR EDUCATION AND REHABILITATION OF THE BLIND AND VISUALLY IMPAIRED (AER)

206 North Washington Street, Suite 320
Alexandria, VA 22314
(703) 548-1884   FAX (703) 683-2926

Administers scholarships for postsecondary students preparing for a career serving individuals who are visually impaired or blind. The Ferrell Scholarship requires that applicants be legally blind. The Telesensory Scholarship requires that applicants be current members of AER. Applications deadline of April 15 in even numbered years.

CHRISTIAN RECORD SERVICES

4444 South 52nd Street
Lincoln, NE 68506
(402) 488-0981   (402) 488-1902 (TT)
FAX (402) 488-7582

Provides financial assistance to students who are legally blind and who are planning to attend an undergraduate college. Applications must be received by April 1 for the following academic year.

COUNCIL OF CITIZENS WITH LOW VISION INTERNATIONAL (CCLVI)

5707 Brockton Drive, #302
Indianapolis, IN 46220-5481
(800) 733-2258   (317) 254-1185
FAX (317) 251-6588

Awards the CCLVI-Telesensory Scholarship of $1,000.00 to an undergraduate student who has low vision but is not totally blind. Application deadline of April 1. The Carl E. Foley Scholarship awards $1,000.00 to a graduate student studying vision rehabilitation at one of five designated institutions.

DOMINICAN COLLEGE OF SAN RAFAEL
Ted Blair, Chair, Department of Music
50 Acacia Avenue
San Rafael, CA 94901-8008
(415) 485-3275

Awards the Rho Barrett Music Scholarship to a student who is legally blind and a music major.

FOUNDATION FOR SCIENCE AND DISABILITY, INC.
Rebecca F. Smith
115 South Brainard Avenue
La Grange, IL 60525

Awards a $1,000.00 scholarship to students entering or continuing in a master's degree program in mathematics, science, medicine, engineering, or computer science. Annual application deadline is December 1.

GEORGE WASHINGTON UNIVERSITY
Disabled Student Services
Rice Hall, Suite 401
2121 Eye Street, NW
Washington, DC 20052

Provides financial assistance to part-time students who are visually impaired or blind through the Barbara Jackman Zuckert Scholarship. Applications must be postmarked by May 30.

NATIONAL FEDERATION OF THE BLIND (NFB)
Attn: Peggy Elliott
814 4th Avenue, Suite 200
Grinnell, IA 50112
(515) 236-3366

RECORDING FOR THE BLIND AND DYSLEXIC (RFB&D)
20 Roszel Road
Princeton, NJ 08540
(800) 221-4792   (609) 452-0606
FAX (609) 987-8116

Scholastic achievement awards for college seniors who are legally blind.

FINANCIAL AID FOR STUDENTS WITH DISABILITIES
HEATH Resource Center
One Dupont Circle, Suite 800
Washington, DC 20036-1193
(800) 544-3284   (202) 939-9320 (V/TT)
FAX (202) 833-4760

Covers the various types of financial aid, such as grants, loans, and work; describes vocational rehabilitation services; and lists organizations which provide scholarships as well as resource directories. P, C, and disk (DOS or Mac); FREE.

FINANCIAL AID FROM THE U.S. DEPARTMENT OF EDUCATION: THE STUDENT GUIDE
Office of Student Financial Assistance
Office of Postsecondary Education
U.S. Department of Education
400 Maryland Avenue, SW
Washington, DC 20202

A booklet describing the various scholarship, loan, and work-study programs funded by the Department of Education; FREE.

Chapter 10

SERVICES FOR VETERANS

Veterans are eligible for a wide range of services from the U.S. Department of Veterans Affairs. Veterans with disabilities are eligible for counseling services and job assistance at Career Development Centers located in VA regional offices. These offices also offer a Vocational Rehabilitation and Counseling Service to help veterans with service connected disabilities receive rehabilitation services and find employment.

All veterans who are legally blind and eligible for VA services are also eligible for Visual Impairment Services Team (VIST) programs. VIST programs are available at most VA Medical Centers throughout the country; they provide a variety of services that help veterans adjust to vision loss, including education, counseling, and self-help groups. When necessary, they refer veterans to Blindness Rehabilitation Centers and Clinics, described below. Contact the local VA Medical Center for more information; if there is no VIST program, the social work department can provide information and make referrals.

AID and Attendance (A & A) status is defined as a level of disability that entitles veterans to a non-service connected VA pension. The VIST coordinator assesses visual functioning and other disabilities to determine A & A status. Veterans are eligible for prosthetic and sensory aids FREE of charge, although more expensive devices are

LIVING WITH LOW VISION: A Resource Guide for People with Sight Loss, Lexington, MA: Resources for Rehabilitation, Copyright 1996

sometimes provided on loan. In October, 1990, the Department of Veterans Affairs issued a legal interpretation that stated that mechanical or electronic equipment, which have been determined by appropriate authorities in the department to aid eligible veterans to "overcome the handicap of blindness," may be furnished by the department.

The Department of Labor, local Veteran Employment Representatives, and Disabled Veteran Outreach Programs also provide services to disabled veterans. The U.S. Department of Education provides funding to institutions of higher education to conduct outreach programs to recruit veterans, including those with disabilities, and to provide counseling and tutoring. Contact the Assistant Secretary for Postsecondary Education, U.S. Department of Education, 400 Maryland Avenue, SW, Washington, D.C. 20202.

DEPARTMENT OF VETERANS AFFAIRS
(800) 827-1000

BLIND REHABILITATION CENTERS

Blind Rehabilitation Centers offer comprehensive blindness rehabilitation programs in a residential setting for veterans who are legally blind and in relatively good health. Enrollment at the centers is free and in some cases, the VA may pay for the veterans' travel costs; the travel clerk at the local VA Medical Center can help determine eligibility.

Participants receive training in orientation and

mobility and skills of daily living; counseling; and a low vision evaluation. Each Blind Rehabilitation Center has an independent living program for those veterans who will be living alone after rehabilitation. The length of the training program depends upon the individual's needs, but usually ranges from eight to sixteen weeks.

There are eight blind rehabilitation centers in the U.S. Regional consultants from each center travel to each VA Medical Center within the region. Contact the VIST coordinator at the local VA Medical Center to obtain more specific information about the program.

AMERICAN LAKE BLIND REHABILITATION CENTER
VA Medical Center (124)
American Lake
Tacoma, WA 98493-5000
(206) 582-8440, extension 6200   FAX (206) 589-4029

CENTRAL BLIND REHABILITATION CENTER
VA Hospital (124)
Hines, IL 60141
(708) 343-7200, extension 3615   FAX (708) 531-7949

EASTERN BLIND REHABILITATION CENTER
VA Medical Center (124)
950 Campbell Avenue
West Haven, CT 06516
(203) 932-5711   FAX (203) 937-3878

PUERTO RICO BLIND REHABILITATION CENTER
VA Medical Center (124)
1 Veterans Plaza
San Juan, PR 00927-5800
(809) 758-7575, extension 4023   FAX (809) 766-6100

SOUTHEASTERN BLIND REHABILITATION CENTER
VA Medical Center (124)
700 South 19th Street
Birmingham, AL 35233
(205) 933-8101   FAX (205) 933-4484

SOUTHWESTERN BLIND REHABILITATION CENTER
VA Medical Center (124)
3601 South 6th Avenue
Tucson, AZ 85723
(520) 629-4643   FAX (520) 629-4642

WACO BLIND REHABILITATION CENTER
VA Medical Center (124)
4800 Memorial Drive
Waco, TX 76711
(817) 752-6581, extension 7487   FAX (817) 752-6581

WESTERN BLIND REHABILITATION CENTER
VA Medical Center (124)
3801 Miranda Boulevard
Palo Alto, CA 94304
(415) 493-5000   FAX (415) 463-4700

VICTORS

Veterans who have experienced vision loss (best corrected acuity of 20/40 or less or significant field loss) but are not legally blind are served by Vision Impairment Centers To Optimize Remaining Sight (VICTORS). VICTORS offers three to five day visual rehabilitation programs which provide low vision evaluations, individual and family counseling, rehabilitation training, and low vision devices.

VICTORS Programs are available at these locations:

NORTHPORT VA MEDICAL CENTER
Building 2 (123)
Northport, NY 11768
(516) 261-4400, extension 2068

VA MEDICAL CENTER
Eye/VICTORS Clinic (112G)
4801 East Linwood Boulevard
Kansas City, MO 64128
(816) 861-4700, extension 7408

VA WEST SIDE MEDICAL CENTER
820 South Damen Avenue
Chicago, IL 60612
(312) 666-6500, extension 3506

OTHER ORGANIZATIONS

BLINDED VETERANS ASSOCIATION (BVA)
477 H Street, NW
Washington, DC 20001-2694
(800) 669-7079   (202) 371-8880
BBS (800) 871-8387

The BVA's field service and outreach employment programs help veterans find rehabilitation services, training, and employment. Offers scholarships to spouses and dependent children of blinded veterans. Membership, $8.00, includes the "BVA Bulletin" in LP and on disc. The BBS, VA ON-LINE, offers information on a variety of benefits for veterans as well as literature on rehabilitation.

DISABLED AMERICAN VETERANS (DAV)
PO Box 14301
Cincinnati, OH 45250-0301
(606) 441-7300   (202) 554-3501 (TT)

DAV National Service Officers advocate for veterans and their families. Provides transportation to VA Medical Centers and emergency relief for veterans with financial crises. Provides scholarships for children of eligible disabled veterans. National DAV Blind Chapter. Membership, $15.00, includes "DAV Magazine," P and C; nonmember subscription, $15.00.

PUBLICATIONS AND TAPES

COORDINATED SERVICES FOR BLINDED VETERANS
Veterans Health Administration
Blind Rehabilitation Service
810 Vermont Avenue, NW
Washington, DC 20420

Describes the services provided at blind rehabilitation centers and clinics. LP, FREE.

FEDERAL BENEFITS FOR VETERANS AND DEPENDENTS
Superintendent of Documents
PO Box 371954
Pittsburgh, PA 15250-7954
(202) 512-1800   FAX (202) 512-2250
telnet federal.bbs.gpo.gov (Port 3001)
BBS (202) 512-1387

Describes the benefits available under federal laws. $2.50

A SUMMARY OF DEPARTMENT OF VETERANS AFFAIRS BENEFITS

Available from any VA regional office; FREE.

TALKING AMERICAN LEGION MAGAZINE
PO Box 1055
Indianapolis, IN 46206

Published monthly on 4-track audiocassette; FREE.

Chapter 11

SERVICES FOR PEOPLE WITH VISION LOSS AND HEARING LOSS

Individuals who are born deaf-blind require special education services and communication training. They often receive their education in special residential schools and may need to be placed in supported employment after they complete their education. Supported employment is paid employment with training and ongoing support provided at the workplace. The U.S. Department of Education provides financial support to state and local education agencies under the "Services for Children with Deaf-Blindness Program," mandated by the Individuals with Disabilities Education Act (IDEA, P.L. 101-476; See Chapter 9, "Services for Children and Adolescents")

Those individuals who become deaf-blind during childhood, adolescence, or as adults often experience difficult emotional adjustment to sudden or unexpected severe loss. Common causes of deaf-blindness in adolescence and beyond include rubella or German measles and Usher syndrome. Usher syndrome is an inherited disorder which causes both retinitis pigmentosa and hearing loss; it may also cause balance problems. Individuals with Type I Usher syndrome have profound hearing loss at birth, retinitis pigmentosa, and balance problems. Individuals with Type II Usher syndrome have moderate to severe hearing loss and retinitis pigmentosa but no balance

LIVING WITH LOW VISION: A Resource Guide for People with Sight Loss, Lexington, MA: Resources for Rehabilitation, Copyright 1996

problems.

With the increasing number of elders in our society, many more individuals are experiencing both hearing loss and vision loss, since both are age-related disabilities. Those individuals who have some sight or hearing may be able to use sign language, speech reading, and assistive devices designed for people who are visually impaired or hearing impaired. In addition, tactile signs, braille, finger spelling, and other communication systems are available for those with no useful vision or hearing.

The number of individuals who are totally deaf and blind is relatively small. Services for these individuals vary from state to state. Contact the state agency that serves individuals who are visually impaired or blind or the general vocational rehabilitation agency. Many states have special agencies that serve people who are deaf or hearing impaired. A special unit that serves individuals who are deaf-blind may exist in any of these three types of agencies. In addition, school systems have special educators for children who are deaf-blind.

AMERICAN ASSOCIATION OF THE DEAF-BLIND (AADB)
814 Thayer Avenue, Room 300
Silver Spring, MD 20910
(301) 588-6545 (TT)   FAX (301) 523-1265

A consumer organization that advocates for coordinated services to individuals who are deaf-blind. Membership, $15.00, includes subscription to quarterly magazine, "The Deaf-Blind American," in LP and B.

CANADIAN DEAF-BLIND AND RUBELLA ASSOCIATION
747 2nd Avenue East, Suite 4
Owen Sound, Ontario N4K 2G9 Canada
(519) 372-1333 (V/TT)   FAX (519) 372-1334

Develops training programs, conferences, and services for individuals who are deaf-blind, their families, and professionals. Eight chapters. Newsletter, "Intervention," published twice a year in P and C. Membership, $15.00.

DB-LINK (NATIONAL INFORMATION CLEARINGHOUSE ON CHILDREN WHO ARE DEAF-BLIND)
345 North Monmouth Avenue
Monmouth, OR 97361
(503) 838-8776   (503) 838-8821 (TT)
FAX (503) 838-8150

Provides information and referral services related to children and youth from birth to age 21 who are deaf-blind. Serves parents, teachers, employers, other professionals, and the public. Produces training manuals on topics ranging from education to independent living. Newsletter, "Deaf-Blind Perspectives," published three times per year, FREE. FREE publications list.

FOUNDATION FIGHTING BLINDNESS
1401 Mt. Royal Avenue
Baltimore, MD 21217
(800) 683-5555   (800) 683-5551 (TT)
(410) 225-9400   (410) 225-9409 (TT)
FAX (410) 225-3936

Provides information about Usher syndrome and makes referrals to Usher Syndrome Self-Help Network. Publishes "Information About Usher Syndrome" and a fact sheet, "Usher Syndrome Backgrounder." LP, FREE.

HEATH RESOURCE CENTER
One Dupont Circle, Suite 800
Washington, DC 20036-1193
(800) 544-3284   (202) 939-9320 (V/TT)
FAX (202) 833-4760

Provides information about the transition from high school to postsecondary education. Publishes newsletter, "Information from HEATH," three times a year. Publishes "Students Who are Deaf or Hard of Hearing in Postsecondary Education," "Career Planning and Employment Strategies," "How to Choose a College: Guide for the Student with a Disability" and "Vocational Rehabilitation

Services: A Postsecondary Student Consumer's Guide."
Publications list and all HEATH publications are FREE in P,
C, and disk (DOS or Mac).

HELEN KELLER NATIONAL CENTER FOR DEAF-BLIND YOUTHS AND ADULTS (HKNC)
111 Middle Neck Road
Sands Point, NY 11050
(516) 944-8900   (516) 944-8637 (TT)
FAX (516) 944-8751

Offers evaluation, rehabilitation, counseling, placement,
and related services through eight regional offices.
Sponsors national network of parents and state and local
parent organizations. Newsletter, "Network Neighbors,"
published three times a year for parents and families of
individuals who are deaf-blind, $15.00. Newsletter for
young persons who are deaf-blind, "HKNC TAC News,"
published three times a year in LP and B, FREE. HKNC's
Specialist to Elderly Deaf-Blind Persons provides services
to professionals in the rehabilitation and aging fields [4455
LBJ Freeway, LB#3, Suite 317, Dallas, TX 75244-5998,
(214) 490-9677].

NATIONAL INFORMATION CENTER ON DEAFNESS
Gallaudet University
800 Florida Avenue, NE
Washington, DC 20002
(202) 651-5051   (202) 651-5052 (TT)
FAX (202) 651-5054

Provides information on education of deaf children, communication, hearing loss and aging, careers working with people who are deaf, and assistive devices. Many inexpensive or FREE publications.

NATIONAL INSTITUTE ON DEAFNESS AND OTHER COMMUNICATIONS DISORDERS INFORMATION CLEARINGHOUSE
1 Communication Avenue
Bethesda, MD 20892-3456
(800) 241-1044   (800) 241-1055 (TT)

Provides information about diseases and disorders of the ear including hereditary and other forms of congenital deafness such as Usher syndrome. FREE publications list.

SELF-HELP FOR HARD OF HEARING PEOPLE (SHHH)
7800 Wisconsin Avenue
Bethesda, MD 20814
(301) 657-2248   (301) 657-2249 (TT)

Educates consumers and professionals about hearing loss. Makes referrals to local chapters, which hold self-help meetings. Holds an annual meeting. Membership, U.S., $15.00; Canada, $20.00; includes subscription to bimonthly magazine "SHHH" and discounts on other publications.

USHER SYNDROME PROJECT/GENETICS

Boys Town National Research Hospital
555 North 30 Street
Omaha, NE 68131
(800) 835-1468 (V/TT)   In NE, (404) 498-6742

Conducts research to locate the gene(s) which cause Usher syndrome. Families are needed to participate in the research.

ABOUT US
Vision Screen Project
5801 Southwood Drive
Bloomington, MN 55437-1739
(612) 831-5522 (V/TT)

Newsletter, written by and for individuals with Usher syndrome II, provides practical information on living with dual sensory loss. Four issue subscription, $14.00. LP, C, and B.

ASSISTIVE DEVICES FOR DEAF-BLIND PERSONS
Canadian National Institute for the Blind
1929 Bayview Avenue
Toronto, Ontario M4G 3E8 Canada
(416) 480-7580   FAX (416) 480-7677

Sells devices by mail. Request "Aids and Devices Catalog," P and B. $20.00, Canadian funds

COPING WITH HEARING LOSS
by Susan V. Rezen and Carl Hausman
Dembner Books/Barricade Books
61 4th Avenue, 3rd Floor
New York, NY 10003-5202
(212) 228-8828

This book discusses the causes of hearing loss, problems experienced by people with hearing loss, solutions for these problems, information about hearing aids, tips on lipreading, and a glossary. $15.95

DEAF-BLINDNESS: NATIONAL ORGANIZATIONS AND RESOURCES
National Library Service for the Blind and Physically Handicapped (NLS)
1291 Taylor Street NW
Washington, DC 20542
(800) 424-8567 or 8572 (Reference Section)
(202) 707-5100   FAX (202) 707-0712

Includes information about rehabilitation, education, recreation services, and sources of assistive devices. LP, FREE

IDENTIFYING VISION AND HEARING PROBLEMS AMONG OLDER PERSONS: STRATEGIES AND RESOURCES
by Martha Bagley
Helen Keller National Center for Deaf-Blind Youth and Adults (HKNC)
111 Middle Neck Road
Sands Point, NY 11050
(516) 944-8900 (V/TT)   FAX (516) 944-8751

A guide for helping elders to identify and cope with dual sensory impairments. P and B. $1.50

I WORK WITH A GUY WHO'S DEAF AND BLIND
Fanlight Productions
47 Halifax Street
Boston, MA 02130
(800) 937-4113   (617) 524-0980
FAX (617) 524-8838

This videotape documents the accommodations a large company made for an employee who is deaf and blind. 11 minutes. Available in open and closed caption formats. Purchase: $125.00; rental: $50.00 a day; $100.00 a week.

LIVING SKILLS: A GUIDE TO INDEPENDENCE FOR INDIVIDUALS WITH DEAF-BLINDNESS
Functional Independence Training, Inc. (FIND)
119 4th Street North, Suite 308
Minneapolis, MN 55401
(612) 333-9102 (V/TT)

Provides instruction for activities of daily living such as eating, personal care, money management, and home care. Includes information on teaching, communications, and family life. LP and B. $35.00

LIVING WITH HEARING LOSS
Resources for Rehabilitation
33 Bedford Street, Suite 19A
Lexington, MA 02173
(617) 862-6455   FAX (617) 861-7517

A LARGE PRINT (18 point bold type) publication that describes organizations and publications that provide assistance to people with hearing loss. Minimum purchase, 25 copies. $1.50 per copy plus shipping and handling. Discounts available for purchases of 100 or more copies. See order form on last page of this book.

RESOURCES FOR ELDERS WITH DISABILITIES
Resources for Rehabilitation
33 Bedford Street, Suite 19A
Lexington, MA 02173
(617) 862-6455   FAX (617) 861-7517

A LARGE PRINT resource directory that describes services and products that elders with disabilities need to function independently. Includes chapters on vision loss, hearing loss, arthritis, diabetes, osteoporosis, Parkinson's disease, falls, and stroke. $43.95 plus $5.00 shipping and handling. See order form on last page of this book.

SOUND AND SIGHT: YOUR SECOND FIFTY YEARS
The Lighthouse, Inc.
111 East 59th Street
New York, NY 10022
(800) 334-5497 (V/TT)   (212) 821-9200
(212) 821-9713 (TT)   FAX (212) 821-9705

A booklet that provides information on age-related hearing and vision loss and lists resources. $5.00. Also available, "Sound and Sight," a brochure which discusses loss of both vision and hearing in older adults. Available in English and Spanish; single copy, FREE.

USHER SYNDROME FAMILY SUPPORT
4918 42nd Avenue South
Minneapolis, MN 55417

Quarterly newsletter for families of individuals with Usher syndrome. U.S., $14.00; foreign, $20.00.

Chapter 12

SPECIAL SERVICES AND PRODUCTS BY EYE DISEASE/CONDITION

AIDS AND VISION LOSS

A number of pathological eye conditions occur in patients with AIDS. The most common of these conditions, cotton wool spots, appear as lesions in the retina and do not usually cause decreased acuity. A more serious effect of AIDS is the cytomegalovirus (CMV), an infection of the retina that can lead to severe visual impairment or blindness if untreated. Two drugs are available to control retinal CMV, ganciclovir and foscarnet, although neither drug offers a cure. Both drugs are administered intravenously, and both may cause serious side effects.

Another possible effect of AIDS on vision is damage to the optic nerve, causing a decrease in contrast sensitivity and color discrimination. Nonviral infections, parasitic diseases, and Kaposi's sarcoma, a cancer that affects the eyelids or conjunctiva, are other conditions related to AIDS.

LIVING WITH LOW VISION: A Resource Guide for People with Sight Loss, Lexington, MA: Resources for Rehabilitation, Copyright 1996

AIDSDRUGS, AIDSTRIALS, and AIDSLINE
National Library of Medicine (NLM)
8600 Rockville Pike
Building 38, Room 2S-10
Bethesda, MD 20894
(800) 272-4787   (301) 496-6095

AIDSDRUGS is a dictionary about new drugs being evaluated to treat AIDS; AIDSTRIALS reports on clinical trials currently underway (including patient eligibility criteria) and those that have been completed; and AIDSLINE contains references to research and policy related to AIDS.

NATIONAL AIDS CLEARINGHOUSE (NAC)
PO Box 6003
Rockville, MD 20849-6003
(800) 458-5231   (800) 243-7012 (TT)
FAX (301) 738-6616

Sponsored by the Centers for Disease Control, NAC provides HIV and AIDS information, referrals, and publications. Spanish and French information specialists are also available. Offers "CDC NAC ONLINE," a bulletin board service, and an AIDS Clinical Trials Information Service at (800) 874-2572 or (800) 243-7012 (TT).

NATIONAL AIDS HOTLINE
(800) 342-2437   (800) 344-7432 (Spanish)
(800) 243-7889 (TT)

A 24 hour hot-line that provides information about HIV

transmission and prevention, HIV testing and treatment, referrals, and educational materials. Special resources are available for minorities and women. Spanish information specialists are bilingual and bicultural. Publications available in English and Spanish, FREE.

NATIONAL INSTITUTE OF ALLERGY AND INFECTIOUS DISEASES (NIAID)
9000 Rockville Pike
Building 31, Room 7A50
Bethesda, MD 20892
(301) 496-5717

Funds federally sponsored AIDS clinical trials. Newsletter, "Dateline: NIAID," FREE.

ALBINISM

Albinism is a hereditary condition in which the amount of pigment in the eyes, hair, and/or skin is deficient. Visual characteristics include decreased acuity, nystagmus (involuntary, rapid eye movements), and photophobia (light sensitivity). Because albinism is a hereditary condition, affected individuals may wish to seek genetic counseling to assist with family planning.

NATIONAL ORGANIZATION FOR ALBINISM AND HYPOPIGMENTATION (NOAH)

1530 Locust Street, #29
Philadelphia, PA 19102
(800) 473-2310   (215) 545-2322

Support organization with chapters and contact people across U.S. Newsletter,"NOAH News," is published in LP, twice a year. Membership, $15.00. Publishes "The Student with Albinism in the Regular Classroom," a book that describes the special needs of children with albinism and suggests adaptations for classroom and nonclassroom activities. LP, $4.00. Also publishes information bulletins on subjects such as African-Americans and albinism, Hermansky-Pudlak Syndrome, social and emotional aspects of albinism, and resources for people with albinism.

CATARACTS

A cataract is a cloudiness or opacity in the lens of the eye which interferes with vision. A common early symptom of cataracts is blurred vision, which may affect reading and night driving. The majority of people with cataracts are over age 60. However, sometimes cataracts are caused by eye inflammations, eye medications, or injury to the eye. The growth of a cataract is usually gradual and painless. A cataract may develop in one eye only or in both eyes at different rates.

A cataract is removed surgically when it seriously affects normal use of vision. Usually an intraocular lens is implanted to replace the natural lens, although contact lenses and cataract glasses have also been used. Cataract surgery is one of the most common surgical procedures performed in the U.S. and has a high success rate. In some cases, however, concurrent eye conditions prohibit cataract surgery or result in less than normal vision.

Cataracts in children are usually hereditary. Congenital cataracts are much more difficult to treat surgically than cataracts in older adults. Some children may benefit from the use of low vision aids, such as reading lenses, telescopic devices, or sunglasses. Individuals with congenital cataracts may wish to seek genetic counseling.

DON'T LOSE SIGHT OF CATARACT
National Eye Institute (NEI)
Building 31, Room 6A32
Bethesda, MD 20892
(301) 496-5248

This booklet discusses causes, treatment, and research. FREE in LP from NEI and C ($2.00) from VISION Foundation, Inc., 818 Mt. Auburn Street, Watertown, MA 02172.

THE PHYSICIAN'S GUIDE TO CATARACTS, GLAUCOMA AND OTHER EYE PROBLEMS
by John Eden, M.D. and the Editors of Consumer Reports Books
Consumer Reports Books
PO Box 10637, Dept. 149310
Des Moines, IA 50336
(800) 500-9759   (515) 237-4903
FAX (515) 284-6713

Written for patients by an ophthalmologist, this book discusses examinations and medical procedures. $18.95

CORNEAL DISORDERS

Keratoconus is a disease in which the cornea thins and develops bulges, causing a decrease in visual acuity. Infections such as herpes simplex virus and trauma to the cornea may also result in vision loss. These conditions may lead to edema (swelling), the development of abnormal blood vessels, and corneal scarring, which prevents light from entering the eye. Antiviral drugs are often successful in treating herpes infections. Corneal transplants are successful in about 80% of all cases, with the remainder of cases rejecting the transplanted tissue or developing additional abnormal blood vessels.

Dry eye or keratoconjunctivitis sicca (KCS) is a condition in which not enough tears are produced; symptoms include burning, itching, sensitive eyes that fatigue easily. It is possible that abnormalities in the cornea contribute to this condition. This condition is also associated with Sjogren's syndrome, a systemic disorder that causes dryness in the mouth and skin as well as the eyes (See "SJOGREN'S SYNDROME" below). Drugs are used in the treatment of this condition with varying degrees of success.

EYE BANK ASSOCIATION OF AMERICA (EBAA)
1001 Connecticut Avenue, NW, Suite 601
Washington, DC 20036-5504
(202) 775-4999   FAX (202) 429-6036

An organization of eye banks in the U.S., Canada, and Mexico which provide tissue for corneal transplants. Funds research projects and promotes eye and tissue donation through posters, brochures, and videotapes.

TISSUE BANKS INTERNATIONAL (TBI)
815 Park Avenue
Baltimore, MD 21201
(410) 752-3800   FAX (410) 727-3843

A network of eye banks throughout the U.S., TBI coordinates the donation of tissue. Provides public information.

DIABETIC RETINOPATHY

Diabetic retinopathy is the major cause of vision loss in young adults. Complications of diabetes that cause vision loss include macular edema, or a build-up of fluid in the central part of the retina, and proliferative retinopathy, the growth of abnormal blood cells which may rupture and then form scar tissue. Diabetic retinopathy is often treated with laser photocoagulation. Sometimes it is necessary to perform a vitrectomy, or surgical removal of blood and scar tissue from the vitreous, in the attempt to restore useful vision.

To manage their diabetes, many people with vision loss use a wide range of adapted equipment such as talking scales and thermometers; syringe magnifiers; and adapted insulin gauges. Several companies have added speech output devices to their blood glucose monitors. It is critical to receive instruction on the use of these meters from a diabetes educator, physician, pharmacist, or sales representative. Contact the Diabetics Division of the National Federation of the Blind (listed below under "ORGANIZATIONS") for an up-to-date list of special equipment. Many hospitals and physicians provide special diabetes education programs to help people with diabetes monitor their own conditions. People with diabetes and vision loss should inquire about training in the use of specially adapted equipment prior to enrolling in these programs.

ORGANIZATIONS

AMERICAN DIABETES ASSOCIATION (ADA)
1660 Duke Street
Alexandria, VA 22314
(800) 232-3472   FAX (703) 836-7439
In Washington, DC area, (703) 549-1500

National office refers callers to local affiliate for education materials.   Membership, U.S., $24.00; Canada, $41.73; includes a subscription to "Diabetes Forecast," a monthly magazine and 10% discount on publications. Many local affiliates offer their own publications, sponsor support groups, and conduct professional training programs.

CANADIAN DIABETES ASSOCIATION (CDA)
15 Toronto Street, Suite 1001
Toronto, Ontario M5C 2E3 Canada
(416) 363-3373

Provides service and education to individuals with diabetes and supports research. Produces a variety of inexpensive educational brochures in English and French.

DIABETICS DIVISION
National Federation of the Blind
811 Cherry Street, Suite 309
Columbia, MO 65201
(314) 875-8911

A national support and information network. Publishes a

quarterly magazine, "Voice of the Diabetic," which includes personal experiences, medical information, recipes, and resources. P and 4-track audiocassette. FREE to members; nonmember subscription, $20.00. Also available, "Resource List: Aids and Appliances," a list of adaptive equipment; LP, C, B; $2.00.

JUVENILE DIABETES FOUNDATION INTERNATIONAL (JDF)
The Diabetes Research Foundation
432 Park Avenue South
New York, NY 10016-8013
(800) 533-2873   (212) 889-7575
FAX (212) 725-7259

JDF Canada:
89 Granton Drive
Richmond Hill, Ontario L4B 2N5 Canada
(800) 668-0274   (905) 889-4171
FAX (905) 889-4209

Raises funds to find the cause, cure, prevention, and treatment of diabetes and its complications. Local chapters provide parent-to-parent counseling and self-help groups for newly diagnosed diabetics and their families. FREE pamphlets and fact sheets. Membership, $25.00, includes subscription to quarterly magazine "Countdown."

NATIONAL DIABETES INFORMATION CLEARINGHOUSE (NDIC)
1 Information Way
Bethesda, MD 20892-3560
(301) 654-3327   http://www.nih.gov/

Clearinghouse for information on all aspects of diabetes. Publishes public and professional education materials and specialized bibliographies. FREE list of publications and many publications are FREE in single copies. Newsletter, "Diabetes Dateline," FREE. Publications available electronically on world wide web home page.

PUBLICATIONS AND TAPES

BUYER'S GUIDE TO DIABETES PRODUCTS
American Diabetes Association (ADA)
1970 Chain Bridge Road
McLean, VA 22109-0592
(800) 232-3472
In Washington, DC area, (703) 549-1500

Compares products from a variety of manufacturers of syringes, insulin pumps, etc. $2.95 plus $3.00 shipping and handling.

DIABETES: CARING FOR YOUR EMOTIONS AS WELL AS YOUR HEALTH

by Jerry Edelwich and Archie Brodsky
Addison Wesley Publishing Company
1 Jacob Way
Reading, MA 01867
(800) 447-2226   (617) 944-3700

Although not specifically written for people with vision loss, this book offers suggestions for adaptations, relationships with medical personnel, family strategies, employment questions, technology, and support groups. $12.45

DIABETES SELF-MANAGEMENT

PO Box 52890
Boulder, CO 80322-2890

A bimonthly magazine that helps people with diabetes manage their conditions independently. Includes articles about special aids, diet, and diabetes education. Six issues, $18.00; 12 issues, $36.00.

DIABETES, VISUAL IMPAIRMENT, AND GROUP SUPPORT: A GUIDEBOOK

by Judith Caditz
The Center for the Partially Sighted
720 Wilshire Boulevard, Suite 200
Santa Monica, CA 90401-1713
(213) 458-3501

Written by a woman with Type I diabetes, this guidebook is designed for individuals with diabetes and vision loss, their families, and professionals. Discusses diabetes mellitus, how it affects vision, psychosocial aspects, diet, adaptive aids, and organizing education/support groups. P and LP, $10.95 plus $2.50 shipping and handling.

DIABETIC RETINOPATHY: INFORMATION FOR PATIENTS
National Eye Institute (NEI)
Building 31, Room 6A32
Bethesda, MD 20892
(301) 496-5248

Discusses the symptoms of diabetic retinopathy; treatment; vitrectomy; and research. Available FREE in LP from NEI and C ($2.00) from VISION Foundation, Inc., 818 Mt. Auburn Street, Watertown, MA 02172.

DON'T BE BLIND TO DIABETES
Lions Clubs International, Public Relations Division
300 22nd Street
Oak Brook, IL 60521
(708) 571-5466   FAX (718) 571-8890

A videotape that discusses the early detection of diabetes, its effect on vision, and interviews with patients and experts in the field. 19 minutes. $19.95 plus $4.85 shipping and handling.

DON'T LOSE SIGHT OF DIABETIC EYE DISEASE: INFORMATION FOR PEOPLE AT RISK
National Eye Institute (NEI)
Building 31, Room 6A32
Bethesda, MD 20892
(301) 496-5248

Describes how diabetes affects the eyes and problems such as cataract, glaucoma, and diabetic retinopathy. Discusses symptoms, diagnosis, and treatment of diabetic retinopathy. FREE in LP from NEI and C ($2.00) from VISION Foundation, Inc., 818 Mt. Auburn Street, Watertown, MA 02172.

EXCHANGE LISTS FOR MEAL PLANNING
American Diabetes Association (ADA)
1970 Chain Bridge Road
McLean, VA 22109-0592
(800) 232-3472
In Washington, DC area, (703) 549-1500

These exchange lists are available in LP, $2.50 plus $3.00 shipping and handling. Also available on 4-track audiocassette from the Diabetics Division, National Federation of the Blind, $2.00; B, $10.00. (See "ORGANIZATIONS" section above.)

KNOW YOUR DIABETES, KNOW YOURSELF
Joslin Diabetes Center
One Joslin Place
Boston, MA 02215
(617) 732-2695   FAX (617) 732-2562

A videotape in which Joslin patients (not actors) talk about the daily issues of diabetes management: using a meal plan; the important roles exercise, monitoring, injections, and foot and eye care play in their lives; and how they manage their disease when sick or traveling. Joslin health professionals discuss the essentials of good diabetes care. 60 minutes. $39.95

LIVING WITH DIABETES ($1.50 per copy)
LIVING WITH DIABETIC RETINOPATHY ($1.75 per copy)
Resources for Rehabilitation
33 Bedford Street, Suite 19A
Lexington, MA 02173
(617) 862-6455   FAX (617) 861-7517

LARGE PRINT (18 point bold type) publications that describe service organizations, publications, and special equipment. Minimum purchase, 25 copies per title. Discounts available for purchases of 100 or more copies. See order form on last page of this book.

SPECIAL EQUIPMENT FOR PEOPLE
WITH VISUAL IMPAIRMENT

Many types of equipment used by individuals with diabetes to monitor and manage their disease are made with LARGE PRINT or speech output. Major distributors of the most commonly used types of equipment are listed below.

BECTON DICKINSON CONSUMER PRODUCTS
Becton Dickinson & Co.
Franklin Lakes, NJ 07417-1880
(800) 365-3321

Magni-Guide with magnification of 2X snaps onto Lilly, Nordisk, and Squibb-Novo insulin bottle caps. May be used with 1 cc and 1/2 cc syringes.

BOEHRINGER MANNHEIM DIAGNOSTICS
9115 Hague Road
Indianapolis, IN 46250-0100
(800) 858-8072

Produces Accu-Chek series of blood glucose monitors that have LARGE PRINT or speech output of blood glucose reading. Call for demonstration from a local representative.

PALCO LABS
8030 Soquel Drive, #104
Santa Cruz, CA 95062-2096
(800) 346-4488   In CA, (408) 476-3151

Manufactures Insul-eze, which magnifies the syringe calibrations, and Load-Matic, which allows users to set the dosage by touch.

SUPREME MEDICAL
27111 Aliso Creek Road, Suite 115
Aliso Viejo, CA 92656
(800) 866-1187   (714) 831-3660
FAX (714) 831-3466

Manufactures Click-Count insulin syringe, which can be filled accurately using touch.

GLAUCOMA

Glaucoma, often called the "sneak thief of sight," is a group of eye diseases which cause increased intraocular pressure, which in turn prevents proper drainage of the fluid in the vitreous and causes damage to the optic disk. Loss in peripheral vision is the first visual symptom of glaucoma. Glaucoma is an age-related disease and occurs with greater frequency in blacks than in whites.

When undiagnosed or left untreated, glaucoma can lead to blindness. Early diagnosis and treatment can prevent much vision loss due to glaucoma. Experts recommend that everyone over the age of 35 have an eye examination with an intraocular pressure check every two years. In addition, the ophthalmologist should examine the optic nerve through dilated pupils. Treatment to control glaucoma includes prescription drugs and surgery.

ORGANIZATIONS

GLAUCOMA FOUNDATION
33 Maiden Lane
New York, NY 10038
(800) 452-8266   (212) 504-1900
FAX (212) 504-1933

Supports research into the causes and treatment of glaucoma. Operates a direct response hot-line. Publishes "Doctor, I Have a Question: A Guide for Patients and Their Families" and "Eye to Eye," a quarterly newsletter; both LP. Single copies, FREE.

GLAUCOMA RESEARCH FOUNDATION
490 Post Street, Suite 1042
San Francisco, CA 94102
(415) 986-3162

Offers public education program; telephone support network; quarterly newsletter, "Gleams," FREE. Operates an eye donor network, which enables researchers to study the eyes donated by glaucoma patients and their families.

NATIONAL GLAUCOMA RESEARCH
American Health Assistance Foundation
15825 Shady Grove Road, Suite 140
Rockville, MD 20850
(800) 437-2423   (301) 948-3244
FAX (301) 258-9454

Toll-free hotline offers current information on research, treatments, and publications.   Quarterly newsletter, "National Glaucoma Research Report," FREE.

PUBLICATIONS AND TAPES

DON'T LOSE SIGHT OF GLAUCOMA: INFORMATION FOR PEOPLE AT RISK
National Eye Institute (NEI)
Building 31, Room 6A32
Bethesda, MD 20892
(301) 496-5248

Brochure that describes open-angle glaucoma, treatment,

and current research. FREE in LP from NEI and C ($2.00) from VISION Foundation, Inc., 818 Mt. Auburn Street, Watertown, MA 02172.

THE PHYSICIAN'S GUIDE TO CATARACTS, GLAUCOMA AND OTHER EYE PROBLEMS
by John Eden, M.D. and the Editors of Consumer Reports Books
Consumer Reports Books
PO Box 10637, Dept. 149310
Des Moines, IA 50336
(800) 500-9759   (515) 237-4903
FAX (515) 284-6713

Written for patients by an ophthalmologist, this book discusses examinations and medical procedures. $18.95

SOME ANSWERS ABOUT GLAUCOMA
American Health Assistance Foundation
15825 Shady Grove Road, Suite 140
Rockville, MD 20850
(800) 437-2423   (301) 948-3244
FAX (301) 258-9474

Describes the major types of glaucoma, risk factors, diagnosis, and treatment; lists helpful references, toll-free numbers, and organizations. LP, FREE.

UNDERSTANDING AND LIVING WITH GLAUCOMA: A REFERENCE GUIDE FOR PATIENTS AND THEIR FAMILIES
Glaucoma Research Foundation
490 Post Street, Suite 1042
San Francisco, CA 94102
(415) 986-3162

Written by a person with glaucoma, this booklet describes living with a chronic health condition. P, English and Spanish. Single copy, FREE. C, $2.00, available from VISION Foundation, Inc., 818 Mt. Auburn Street, Watertown, MA 02172.

MACULAR DEGENERATION

Macular degeneration may be caused by any of a number of eye conditions that result in the deterioration of the cells in the macula, which is the central part of the retina. Macular degeneration is most common among elders; however, it can also affect young people, due to hereditary factors or injury. The term "age-related" is used to describe the type of macular degeneration which occurs most frequently among individuals age 50 or older. Early detection of macular degeneration is aided by the use of an Amsler Grid, available from ophthalmologists or optometrists. Individuals who detect signs of distortion in their vision should see an ophthalmologist immediately.

The most common form of age-related macular degeneration, the drusenoid or "dry" form, cannot be treated. The neovascular or "wet" form involves the development of abnormal blood vessels and usually causes more severe impairment than the "dry" form. Since the macula is the portion of the retina that is responsible for reading, loss of function in this part of the eye can have a major effect on carrying out routine activities.

The "wet" form may sometimes be treated by laser, depending upon the location of the lesion and a variety of other factors. However, it is common for individuals who have had neovascular membranes treated by laser to develop additional membranes in the same eye.

New treatments for neovascular membranes are currently being investigated by a variety of researchers. Among these treatments is surgical removal of the membranes. To date, studies of this technique, which are based on extremely small samples of patients, have produced conflicting results, but several studies have not found the treatment to be beneficial for people with age-related macular degeneration. Other investigations include the effects of light on age-related eye changes and the use of vitamin supplements as a measure to prevent macular degeneration.

Best disease or vitelliform macular degeneration is a hereditary form of the disease passed on by dominant genes and is usually detected in a child's early years. Stargardt's disease, also known as fundus flavimaculatus or juvenile macular dystrophy, is passed on by recessive genes and is usually detected in the teen-age years.

ASSOCIATION FOR MACULAR DISEASES
210 East 64th Street
New York, NY 10021
(212) 605-3719

Membership organization which holds meetings in New York City area; helps to start chapters in other geographical areas; and arranges special programs in other parts of the country. Provides public education, support, and hot-line for macular degeneration patients. Membership, $20.00, includes newsletter.

FOUNDATION FIGHTING BLINDNESS
1401 Mt. Royal Avenue
Baltimore, MD 21217
(800) 683-5555   (800) 683-5551 (TT)
(410) 225-9400   (410) 225-9409 (TT)
FAX (410) 225-3936

Local chapters, support groups, and information centers for people with macular degeneration, retinitis pigmentosa, and other retinal diseases. Supports research and retina donor program and makes referrals to retina specialists. Provides public and professional education materials and quarterly newsletter, "Fighting Blindness News," LP, C, and B; FREE.

MACULAR DEGENERATION INTERNATIONAL

2968 West Ina Road, #106
Tucson, AZ 85741
(800) 393-7634   (607) 797-2525
FAX (607) 797-2525

Support network for individuals with early or late onset macular degeneration. Membership, $25.00, includes newsletter and resource guide.

PUBLICATIONS AND TAPES

COPING WITH THE DIAGNOSIS OF SIGHT LOSS

Resources for Rehabilitation
33 Bedford Street, Suite 19A
Lexington, MA 02173
(617) 862-6455   FAX (617) 861-7517

An audiocassette in which three consumers, one of whom has macular degeneration, discuss their reactions and experiences when told that they were losing their vision. $12.00 plus $3.00 shipping and handling.

DON'T LOSE SIGHT OF AGE-RELATED MACULAR DEGENERATION: INFORMATION FOR PEOPLE AT RISK

National Eye Institute (NEI)
Building 31, Room 6A32
Bethesda, MD 20892
(301) 496-5248

A brochure that discusses symptoms of age-related

macular degeneration, treatment, and research. FREE in LP from NEI and C, $2.00, from VISION Foundation, Inc., 818 Mt. Auburn Street, Watertown, MA 02172.

I KEEP FIVE PAIRS OF GLASSES IN A FLOWER POT
by Henrietta Levner
National Association for the Visually Handicapped (NAVH)
22 West 21st Street
New York, NY 10010
(212) 889-3141

This booklet describes an older woman's experience learning to live with low vision due to macular degeneration. LP. Members, $2.00; nonmembers, $3.00.

LIVING WITH AGE-RELATED MACULAR DEGENERATION
Resources for Rehabilitation
33 Bedford Street, Suite 19A
Lexington, MA 02173
(617) 862-6455   FAX (617) 861-7517

A LARGE PRINT (18 point bold type) publication that describes service organizations and publications that help people with macular degeneration. Minimum purchase, 25 copies. $1.25 per copy plus shipping and handling. Discounts available for purchases of 100 or more copies. See order form on last page of this book.

LOOK OUT FOR ANNIE
The Lighthouse, Inc.
111 East 59th Street
New York, NY 10022
(800) 334-5497 (V/TT) (212) 821-9200
(212) 821-9713 (TT)   FAX (212) 821-9705

This videotape portrays an older woman with macular degeneration and her interactions with her family, friends, and other elders at the senior center. Discussion guide included. $25.00, VHS or beta format.

OUT OF THE CORNER OF MY EYE: LIVING WITH VISION LOSS IN LATER LIFE
by Nicolette Pernod Ringgold
American Foundation for the Blind (AFB)
c/o American Book Center
Brooklyn Navy Yard, Building No. 3
Brooklyn, NY 11205
(718) 852-9873   FAX (718) 935-9647

Written by a woman who became legally blind in her late 70's due to macular degeneration, this book offers practical advice and encouragement for elders with vision loss. LP and C, $16.95 plus $3.50 shipping and handling.

MONOCULAR VISION

Monocular vision is most frequently caused by trauma or diseases that require removal of an eye. Ocular trauma from sports injuries, fireworks, lawnmower accidents, and automobile accidents may result in monocular vision. Retinoblastoma, a cancer that requires removal of the eye, is the most common primary tumor of the eye in children. In adults, ocular melanoma is the most common primary eye cancer.

When an eye is surgically removed (enucleated), it is usually replaced by a prosthesis (artificial eye). An ocularist is a professional who works with the ophthalmologist in prescribing, selecting, and fitting a prosthesis. Plastic surgery may be required to repair the eye socket and surrounding tissue. A properly fitted prosthesis will allow satisfactory eye movement and appear as similar to the remaining eye as possible.

A major functional limitation of monocular vision is the loss of depth perception. The visual field is reduced and visual processing becomes disorganized. Individuals must learn to move more slowly, to move their heads to compensate for visual field loss, and to develop techniques for judging distance. Optical aids such as magnifiers and monocular telescopes, LARGE PRINT, and improved lighting are all useful in adapting to monocular vision. Individuals with monocular vision should wear safety glasses to protect their remaining vision.

A SINGULAR VIEW: THE ART OF SEEING WITH ONE EYE
by Frank B. Brady
Frank B. Brady Author/Publisher
PO Box 4653
Annapolis, MD 21403
(410) 263-8388

Describes the author's experience adjusting to monocular vision. Includes suggestions for improving visual function and techniques for everyday tasks. Adaptive aids are also discussed. $15.00

SINGULAR VISION OUTREACH (SVOR)
PO Box 1451
Maryland Heights, MO 63043
(314) 453-9905

Assists individuals adjusting to monocular vision and their families through information and referral, support, and consultation. Educates the general public about eye safety and works with health professionals. Publishes newsletter, "An Eye on the Future," and "Driving Tips for Monocular Individuals," FREE. Membership, individual $15.00; family, $25.00.

MULTIPLE SCLEROSIS

Multiple sclerosis (MS) is a chronic disease which affects the central nervous system. Individuals with multiple sclerosis generally experience attacks and remissions of symptoms. The visual symptoms may include blurred vision in one eye, double vision, or nystagmus. Visual symptoms are often transitory and improve or clear within a few months. Inflammation of the optic nerve (neuritis) causes loss of vision. If the muscles of the eye are weakened by multiple sclerosis, the individual cannot focus and experiences double vision (diplopia). Double vision may occur during an exacerbation of the disease and disappear during remission. Cortisone is often used to treat optic neuritis and double vision. Nystagmus is an involuntary rapid eye movement; it interferes with focusing and may cause dizziness.

LIVING WITH MULTIPLE SCLEROSIS: A NEW HANDBOOK FOR FAMILIES
by Robert Shuman and Janice Schwartz
Macmillan Publishing Company
201 West 103rd Street
Indianapolis, IN 46290
(800) 428-5331

Discusses the role of the family, adolescents with MS, and lists resources. $10.00 plus $3.00 shipping and handling.

MULTIPLE SCLEROSIS SOCIETY OF CANADA
250 Bloor Street, East, Suite 1000
Toronto, Ontario M4W 3P9 Canada
(416) 922-6065   In Canada, (800) 268-7582
FAX (416) 922-7538

A national membership organization that funds research,

promotes public education, encourages social action on behalf of individuals with multiple sclerosis, and produces many public and professional publications in English and French. The "ASK MS Information System" database of articles on topics such as treatment, research, and social services, is available to people with multiple sclerosis, family members, and health care professionals. Regional divisions and chapters located throughout Canada. National membership, $12.00, Canadian funds; includes newsletter "MS Canada." Membership is FREE to individuals with multiple sclerosis who live in Canada.

NATIONAL MULTIPLE SCLEROSIS SOCIETY
733 Third Avenue
New York, NY 10017-3288
(800) 344-4867
(212) 986-3240   FAX (212) 986-7981

Offers information and referral, counseling services, physician referrals, advocacy, discount prescription and health care products program, and assistance in obtaining adaptive equipment. Regional affiliates throughout the U.S. Publishes a series of "Fact & Issues" articles, including "Insight into Eyesight" (LP); FREE. Membership, $20.00, includes LP magazine, "Inside MS," published three times a year. Individuals with multiple sclerosis may receive a courtesy membership if they are unable to pay.

TALKING BOOKS FOR PEOPLE WITH PHYSICAL DISABILITIES
National Library Service for the Blind and Physically Handicapped (NLS)
1291 Taylor Street, NW
Washington, DC 20542
(800) 424-8567 or 8572 (Reference Section)
(202) 707-5100   FAX (202) 707-0712

Describes the eligibility requirements for individuals with physical disabilities including multiple sclerosis. FREE.

RETINITIS PIGMENTOSA

Retinitis pigmentosa (RP) is an inherited eye disease which causes degeneration of the retina's photoreceptor cells (called rods and cones). Night blindness and peripheral vision loss are symptoms of rod cell degeneration. If cone cells are affected, the individual may experience decreased central vision and loss of color vision. Retinitis pigmentosa is difficult to diagnose, but as it progresses, retinal changes may be detected by electroretinogram (ERG) and visual field and visual function tests. The progression of symptoms is unpredictable and varies with the genetic forms of the disease. Recent clinical trials sponsored by the National Eye Institute indicate that a 15,000 IU vitamin A supplement, in the form of vitamin A palmitate, may slow the annual decline of retinal function by an average of 20 percent. The trials also found that high doses of vitamin E should be avoided.

Usher syndrome is an inherited disorder which causes both retinitis pigmentosa and hearing loss; it may also cause balance problems. Individuals with Type I Usher syndrome have profound hearing loss at birth, retinitis pigmentosa, and balance problems. Individuals with Type II Usher syndrome have moderate to severe hearing loss and retinitis pigmentosa but no balance problems. (See Chapter 11, "Services for People with Vision Loss and Hearing Loss")

ORGANIZATIONS

ALLIANCE OF GENETIC SUPPORT GROUPS
35 Wisconsin Circle, Suite 440
Chevy Chase, MD 20815
(800) 336-4363   (301) 652-5553
FAX (301) 654-0171

A coalition of support groups for consumers and professionals concerned with genetic diseases. Sponsors national conferences. Membership, individuals, $20.00; organizations, $50.00; includes monthly bulletin, "ALERT."

FOUNDATION FIGHTING BLINDNESS
1401 Mt. Royal Avenue
Baltimore, MD 21217
(800) 683-5555   (800) 683-5551 (TT)
(410) 225-9400   (410) 225-9409 (TT)
FAX (410) 225-3936

Supports research, retina donor program, and national RP registry. Makes referrals to retina specialists. Provides public and professional education materials and quarterly newsletter, "Fighting Blindness News," LP, C, and B; FREE. Local chapters, support groups, and information centers. Publishes "Information about RP and Allied Retinal Degenerative Diseases," "The RP Backgrounder," "Information About Usher Syndrome," and "Usher Syndrome Backgrounder," in LP; FREE.

RP INTERNATIONAL
PO Box 900
Woodland Hills, CA 91365
(800) 344-4877   (818) 992-0500
FAX (818) 992-3265

Information clearinghouse; public education materials. Provides counseling, referrals, and supports research. Newsletter, "The Night Lighter," LP; FREE.

TEXAS ASSOCIATION OF RP (TARP)
PO Box 8388
Corpus Christi, TX 78468-8388
(512) 852-8515

Clearinghouse for RP information; quarterly newsletter, "RP Messenger," provides support and information for RP patients.

USHER SYNDROME PROJECT/GENETICS
Boys Town National Research Hospital
555 North 30 Street
Omaha, NE 68131
(800) 835-1468 (V/TT)   In NE, (404) 498-6742

Conducts research to locate the gene(s) which cause Usher syndrome. Families are needed to participate in the research.

THE BUSINESS OF LIVING PUBLICATIONS
by Dorothy H. Stiefel
PO Box 8388
Corpus Christi, TX 78468-8388
(512) 852-3993

A series of booklets about dealing with retinitis pigmentosa and vision loss: "Dealing with the Threat of Loss" focuses on aspects of daily living with RP from diagnosis to coping. Bold-face type, $4.50; C: English, $6.00; Spanish or French, $7.50. Add postage and handling, U.S., $2.00; Canada, $3.00.

"The 'Madness' of Usher's: Coping with Vision and Hearing Loss" describes the author's experience in living with Type II Usher syndrome. Bold-face type, $7.50; C, $12.50. Add postage and handling, U.S., $2.00; Canada, $3.00

"Stress and Well-Being" offers ways to deal with the stress of everyday living which is intensified for an individual with inconsistent vision. Bold-face type: $4.50; audiocassette: English only, $6.00. Add postage and handling, U.S., $2.00; Canada, $3.00.

COPING WITH THE DIAGNOSIS OF SIGHT LOSS
Resources for Rehabilitation
33 Bedford Street, Suite 19A
Lexington, MA 02173
(617) 862-6455   FAX (617) 861-7517

An audiocassette in which three consumers, one of whom has retinitis pigmentosa, discuss their reactions and experiences when told that they were losing their vision. $12.00 plus $3.00 shipping and handling.

HOW DO I DO THIS WHEN I CAN'T SEE WHAT I'M DOING? INFORMATION PROCESSING FOR THE VISUALLY DISABLED
by Gerald Jahoda
Superintendent of Documents
PO Box 371954
Pittsburgh, PA 15250-7954
(202) 512-1800   FAX (202) 512-2250
telnet federal.bbs.gpo.gov (Port 3001)
BBS (202) 512-1387

The author, who is blind due to retinitis pigmentosa, describes his own experiences in developing new ways to conduct everyday activities at home and at work. LP. Available in U.S. Government Bookstores. S/N 030-000-00248-2 $5.50. Also available on 4-track audiocassette from National Library Service for the Blind and Physically Handicapped regional libraries, RC 36212.

HOW TO SURVIVE LOSING SIGHT
by Helen Harris
RP International
PO Box 900
Woodland Hills, CA 91365
(800) 344-4877   (818) 992-0500

Written by a woman with retinitis pigmentosa, this booklet provides practical information about living with this degenerative retinal disease. P, $11.95; C, $9.95; plus $3.95 shipping and handling.

THE INHERITANCE OF RP AND ALLIED RETINAL DEGENERATIVE DISEASES
by Jill C. Hennessey
Foundation Fighting Blindness
1401 Mt. Royal Avenue
Baltimore, MD 21217
(800) 683-5555   (800) 683-5551 (TT)
(410) 225-9400   (410) 225-9409 (TT)
FAX (410) 225-3936

A booklet that describes the basic genetics and inheritance patterns of retinitis pigmentosa, including autosomal dominant, autosomal recessive, and x-linked (sex linked). Defines allied retinal degenerative diseases such as Best disease, Stargardt disease, choroideremia, and Usher syndrome. Glossary. Lists RP Research Centers. LP, C, and B; FREE.

USHER'S SYNDROME: WHAT IT IS, HOW TO COPE, AND HOW TO HELP
by Earlene Duncan, Hugh T. Prickett, Dan Finkelstein, McCay Vernon, and Toni Hollingsworth
Charles C. Thomas, Publisher
2600 South First Street
Springfield, IL 62794-9265
(800) 258-8980   (217) 789-8980
FAX (217) 789-9130

Includes interviews with individuals with Usher syndrome, psychological adjustment to the diagnosis, and educational and vocational concerns. Hardcover, $32.95; softcover, $18.95; plus $5.50 shipping and handling.

RETINOPATHY OF PREMATURITY
See Chapter 9, "Services for Children and Adolescents"

SJOGREN'S SYNDROME

Sjogren's Syndrome is a chronic condition characterized by dryness of the eyes, mouth, and skin. It accompanies rheumatic disease, often rheumatoid arthritis. Artificial tears and eye drops, mouth rinses and fluids, and moisturizing lotions are used to treat this syndrome.

NATIONAL SJOGREN'S SYNDROME ASSOCIATION
3201 West Evans Drive
Phoenix, AZ 85023
(800) 395-6772   (602) 516-0787

Provides information to patients and professionals through support groups and conferences throughout the U.S. Membership, $20.00, includes quarterly Patient Education Series and newsletter, "Sjogren's Digest." Publishes "Sjogren's Syndrome: The Sneaky Arthritis." U.S., $12.50; foreign, $14.00.

SJOGREN'S SYNDROME FOUNDATION
333 North Broadway
Jericho, NY 11753
(800) 475-4736   (516) 933-6365
FAX (516) 933-6368

Support organization with chapters in U.S., Canada, and abroad. Membership, U.S., $25.00; Canada, $30.00; includes monthly newsletter, "The Moisture Seekers." Publishes "The Sjogren's Syndrome Handbook," a guide for living more comfortably with this chronic illness. Members, $19.95; nonmembers, $24.95; plus $2.50 shipping and handling; shipping to Canada, $7.00.

STROKE RELATED VISION LOSS

Individuals who have had a stroke may lose some of their visual field. A loss of right visual field in both eyes is called "right hemiplegia;" loss of left visual field in both eyes is called "left hemiplegia." Individuals with hemiplegia must learn to turn their heads to compensate. Some individuals find that using a patch over one eye helps to reduce spatial problems due to hemiplegia.

ORGANIZATIONS

HEART AND STROKE FOUNDATION OF CANADA
160 George Street, Suite 200
Ottawa, Ontario K1N 9M2 Canada
(613) 237-4361

Conducts research and provides professional and public education through provincial divisions and chapters. FREE publications list.

NATIONAL STROKE ASSOCIATION
8400 East Orchard Road, Suite 1000
Englewood, CO 80111
(800) 787-6537   (303) 771-1700
(303) 771-1887 (TT)   FAX (303) 771-1886

Assists individuals with stroke and educates their families, physicians, and the general public about stroke. Membership, $10.00, includes quarterly newsletter, "Be Stroke Smart." Also available, "The Road Ahead: A Stroke Recovery Guide." $14.50

STROKE CONNECTION
American Heart Association (AHA)
7272 Greenville Avenue
Dallas, TX 75231
(800) 553-6321

Coordinates a network of more than 800 stroke clubs and groups. Publishes bimonthly newsletter, "Stroke Connection," $8.00; a courtesy subscription is available to any stroke survivor unable to pay. The American Heart Association promotes research and education and publishes public education brochures. Publications that discuss stroke-related vision loss include "Recovering from a Stroke" and "Strokes - A Guide for the Family." Single copies, FREE; also available from affiliates.

PUBLICATIONS

AFTER A STROKE
Resources for Rehabilitation
33 Bedford Street, Suite 19A
Lexington, MA 02173
(617) 862-6455   FAX (617) 861-7517

A LARGE PRINT (18 point bold type) publication that includes information on how to obtain services; organizations that serve people who have had strokes; publications; and aids that help people who have had strokes. Minimum purchase, 25 copies. $1.50 per copy plus shipping and handling. Discounts available for purchases of 100 or more copies. See order form on last page of this book.

RESOURCES FOR ELDERS WITH DISABILITIES
Resources for Rehabilitation
33 Bedford Street, Suite 19A
Lexington, MA 02173
(617) 862-6455   FAX (617) 861-7517

A **LARGE PRINT** resource directory that describes services and products that help elders with disabilities to function independently. Includes chapters on stroke, vision loss, hearing loss, arthritis, diabetes, Parkinson's disease, falls, and osteoporosis. $43.95 plus $5.00 shipping and handling.

APPENDIX A
MAIN OFFICES OF STATE AGENCIES
THAT SERVE INDIVIDUALS
WHO ARE VISUALLY IMPAIRED OR BLIND

To learn the address of the state agency nearest you, contact the main office listed below or the information operator for the state government. Toll-free telephone numbers usually operate only within the state.

ALABAMA
Department of Rehabilitation Services
Services for the Deaf and Blind
2129 East South Boulevard
PO Box 11586
Montgomery, AL 36111-0586
(334) 281-8780 (V/TT)   FAX (334) 281-1973

ALASKA
Office of Vocational Rehabilitation
801 West 10th Street, Suite 200
Juneau, AK 99801
(800) 478-2815   (907) 465-2814 (V/TT)
FAX (907) 465-2856

ARIZONA
State Services for the Blind
1789 West Jefferson, 2nd Floor, NW
Phoenix, AZ 85007
(602) 542-3332   (602) 542-6049 (TT)
FAX (602) 542-3778

ARKANSAS
Division of Services for the Blind
411 Victory Street, PO Box 3237
Little Rock, AR 72201
(800) 482-5850, extension 324-9270
(501) 324-9270　　　　　　FAX (501) 324-9280
(501) 324-9271 (TT)

CALIFORNIA
Department of Rehabilitation
Services for the Blind and Visually Impaired
830 K Street Mall, LL10
Sacramento, CA 95814
(916) 445-9040　　　　　　FAX (916) 327-6919

COLORADO
Rehabilitation Center for the Blind and Visually Impaired
2211 West Evans Avenue
Denver, CO 80223
(303) 937-1226 (V/TT)　　　FAX (303) 934-6854

CONNECTICUT
Services for the Blind
170 Ridge Road
Wethersfield, CT 06109
(800) 842-4510　　　　　　(203) 249-8525 (V/TT)
FAX (203) 278-6920

DELAWARE
Division for the Visually Impaired
1901 North Dupont Highway
Biggs Building
Newcastle, DE 19720
(302) 577-4731   FAX (302) 577-4758

DISTRICT OF COLUMBIA
Visual Impairment Section
Rehabilitation Services Administration
605 G Street NW, 9th Floor
Washington, DC 20001
(202) 727-0907 (V/TT)   FAX (202) 727-1707

FLORIDA
Division of Blind Services
Koger Executive Center
2540 Executive Center Circle, West
Tallahassee, FL 32399
(800) 342-1828   (904) 488-1330 (V/TT)
FAX (904) 487-1804

GEORGIA
Division of Rehabilitation Services
2801 R. N. Martin Street
Wagonworks Building
East Point, GA 30344
(800) 359-1112   (404) 669-3450 (V/TT)
FAX (404) 669-2922

GUAM
Department of Vocational Rehabilitation
PO Box 2950
Agana, Guam 96910
475-4646 (for international calls, dial 671 for country code)
FAX (671) 477-2892

HAWAII
Department of Human Services
Services for the Blind Branch
1901 Bachelot Street
Honolulu, HI 96817
(808) 586-5269 (V/TT)   FAX (808) 586-5288

IDAHO
Commission for the Blind
341 West Washington
Boise, ID 83720-0012
(800) 542-8688   (208) 334-3220
FAX (208) 334-2963

ILLINOIS
Bureau of Blind Services
Illinois Department of Rehabilitation Services
623 East Adams Street
PO Box 19429
Springfield, IL 62794-9429
(800) 275-3677   (217) 782-2093
(217) 785-9328 (TT)   FAX (217) 524-1235

INDIANA
Services for the Blind and Visually Impaired
402 West Washington Street, Room W453
PO Box 7083
Indianapolis, IN 46207-7083
(800) 545-7763   (317) 232-1433

IOWA
Department for the Blind
524 Fourth Street
Des Moines, IA 50309
(800) 362-2587   (515) 281-7999
(515) 281-1355 (TT)   FAX (515) 281-1263

KANSAS
Division of Services for the Blind
Biddle Building, 2nd Floor
300 Southwest Oakley Street
Topeka, KS 66606-1995
(913) 296-4454 (V/TT)   FAX (913) 296-0511

KENTUCKY
Department for the Blind
PO Box 757
Frankfort, KY 40602-0757
(800) 321-6668   (502) 564-4754
(502) 564-2929 (TT)   FAX (502) 564-2951

LOUISIANA
LA Rehabilitation Services
8225 Florida Boulevard
Baton Rouge, LA 70806
(800) 256-1523   (800) 543-2099 (TT)
(504) 925-4131   FAX (504) 925-4184

MAINE
Office of Rehabilitation Services
Division for Blind and Visually Impaired
35 Anthony Avenue
Augusta, ME 04333-0150
(800) 332-1003 (V/TT)   (207) 625-5321 (V/TT)
(207) 624-5318   FAX (207) 624-5302

MARYLAND
Division of Rehabilitation Services
Maryland Rehabilitation Center
2301 Argonne Drive
Baltimore, MD 21218
(410) 554-9405   (410) 554-9411 (TT)
FAX (410) 554-9412

MASSACHUSETTS
Commission for the Blind
88 Kingston Street
Boston, MA 02111
(800) 392-6450   (800) 392-6556 (TT)
(617) 727-5550   FAX (617) 727-5960

MICHIGAN
Commission for the Blind
201 North Washington, PO Box 30015
Lansing, MI 48909
(800) 292-4200   (517) 373-2062
(517) 373-4025 (TT)   FAX (517) 335-5140

MINNESOTA
State Services for the Blind
2200 University Avenue, West, Suite 240
St. Paul, MN 55114-1840
(800) 652-9000   (612) 642-0500
(612) 642-0506 (TT)   FAX (612) 649-5927

MISSISSIPPI
Vocational Rehabilitation for the Blind
PO Box 5314
Jackson, MS 39296-5314
(601) 364-2700   FAX (601) 364-2677

MISSOURI
Rehabilitation Services for the Blind
619 East Capitol Avenue
Jefferson City, MO 65101
(314) 751-4249   (800) 735-2966 (TT)
FAX (314) 751-4984

MONTANA
Visual Services Division
111 Sanders Street, PO Box 4210
Helena, MT 59604-4210
(406) 444-2590 (V/TT)   FAX (406) 444-3632

NEBRASKA
Division of Rehabilitation Services for the Visually Impaired
4600 Valley Road
Lincoln, NE 68510-4844
(402) 471-2891 (V/TT)   FAX (402) 471-3009

NEVADA
Bureau of Services to the Blind and Visually Impaired
Capitol Complex
505 East King, Room 501
Carson City, NV 89710
(702) 687-4444   (702) 687-4440 (TT)
FAX (702) 687-5980

NEW HAMPSHIRE
Services for Blind and Visually Impaired
78 Regional Drive, Building 2
Concord, NH 03301-8508
(800) 299-1647   (603) 271-3537
(603) 271-3471 (TT)   FAX (603) 271-3816

NEW JERSEY
Commission for the Blind and Visually Impaired
153 Halsey Street, 6th Floor
PO Box 47017
Newark, NJ 07101
(800) 962-1233   (201) 648-3333
(201) 648-4559 (TT)   FAX (201) 648-7364

NEW MEXICO
Commission for the Blind
PERA Building, Room 553
Santa Fe, NM 87503
(505) 827-4479   FAX (505) 827-4475

NEW YORK
Commission for the Blind and Visually Handicapped
Mailing address:
40 North Pearl Street
Albany, NY 12243
Office:
Twin Towers, 1 Commerce Plaza, Room 724
Albany, NY 12210
(518) 474-6812   (518) 474-7672 (TT)
FAX (518) 486-5819

NORTH CAROLINA
Division of Services for the Blind
309 Ashe Avenue
Raleigh, NC 27606
(919) 733-9822   (919) 733-9700 (TT)
FAX (919) 733-9769

NORTH DAKOTA
Office of Vocational Rehabilitation
400 East Broadway Avenue, Suite 303
Bismarck, ND 58501-4038
(800) 472-2622   (328) 224-3999
(701) 328-3975 (TT)   FAX (328) 224-3976

OHIO
Bureau of Services for the Visually Impaired
400 East Campus View Boulevard
Columbus, OH 43235-4604
(800) 282-4536 (V/TT)   (614) 438-1255
FAX (614) 438-1257

OKLAHOMA
Visual Services
2409 North Kelley Street, 4th Floor Annex
PO Box 36659
Oklahoma City, OK 73136
(800) 845-8476   (800) 833-8973 (TT)
(405) 522-6006   (405) 424-2794 (TT)
FAX (405) 427-5565

OREGON
Commission for the Blind
535 Southeast 12th Avenue
Portland, OR 97214
(503) 731-3221   (503) 731-3224 (TT)
FAX (503) 731-3230

PENNSYLVANIA
Office for Blindness and Visual Services
1401 North Seventh Street, First Floor, PO Box 2675
Harrisburg, PA 17105
(800) 622-2842   (717) 787-6176
(717) 787-6176 (TT)   FAX (717) 787-3210

PUERTO RICO
Vocational Rehabilitation Program
PO Box 19118
San Juan, PR 00919-1118
(809) 725-1792   FAX (809) 721-6286

RHODE ISLAND
State Services for the Blind and Visually Impaired
40 Fountain Street
Providence, RI 02903
(800) 752-0888   (401) 277-2300
(401) 277-3010 (TT)   FAX (401) 277-1328

SOUTH CAROLINA
Commission for the Blind
1430 Confederate Avenue
Columbia, SC 29201
(800) 922-2222   (803) 734-7520
FAX (803) 734-7885

SOUTH DAKOTA
Division of Service to Visually Impaired
East Highway 34, 500 East Capitol
Pierre, SD 57501-5070
(800) 265-9684   (605) 773-4644
(605) 773-5990 (TT)   FAX (605) 773-5483

TENNESSEE
Services for the Blind
Citizens Plaza Building, 11th Floor
400 Deaderick Street
Nashville, TN 37248-6200
(800) 270-1349   (615) 313-4914
(615) 313-6601 (TT)   FAX (615) 741-6508

TEXAS
Commission for the Blind
4800 North Lamar, Suite 100
Austin, TX 78756
(800) 252-5204   (512) 459-2544
(512) 459-2546 (TT)   FAX (512) 459-2685

UTAH
Division of Services for the Visually Impaired
309 East 100th South
Salt Lake City, UT 84111
(800) 284-1823   (801) 533-9393 (V/TT)
FAX (801) 538-0437

VERMONT
Bureau for the Blind and Visually Handicapped
Osgood Building
103 South Main Street
Waterbury, VT 05671-2304
(802) 241-2210 (V/TT)   FAX (802) 241-3359

VIRGINIA
Department for the Visually Handicapped
397 Azalea Avenue
Richmond, VA 23227
(800) 622-2155   (804) 371-3140 (V/TT)
FAX (804) 371-3351

WASHINGTON
Department of Services for the Blind
1400 South Evergreen Park Drive, Suite 100
Olympia, WA 98504-0933
(800) 552-7103   (360) 586-1224
(360) 586-6437 (TT)   FAX (360) 586-7627

WEST VIRGINIA
Division of Rehabilitation Services
State Capitol Complex
Charleston, WV 25305
(800) 642-3021   (304) 766-4600
(304) 766-4965 (TT)   FAX (304) 766-4961

WISCONSIN
Office for the Blind
2917 International Lane
PO Box 7852
Madison, WI 53707
(608) 266-5600   (608) 266-9599 (TT)
FAX (608) 267-3657

WYOMING
Services for the Visually Handicapped
Room 144 Hathaway Building
Cheyenne, WY 82002
(307) 777-7274; 777-7256   (307) 777-6221 (TT)
FAX (307) 777-6234

APPENDIX B

DIVISION OFFICES OF
THE CANADIAN NATIONAL INSTITUTE FOR THE BLIND

NATIONAL LIBRARY
1929 Bayview Avenue
Toronto, Ontario M4G 3E8
(800) 268-8818   (416) 480-7520
FAX (416) 480-7700   e-mail cnib-library@immedia.ca

ALBERTA - N.W.T.
12010 Jasper Avenue
Edmonton, Alberta T5K 0P3
(800) 365-2642   (403) 488-4871
FAX (403) 482-0017

BRITISH COLUMBIA - YUKON
5055 Joyce Street, #100
Vancouver, British Columbia V5R 6B2
(604) 431-2121   (604) 431-2131 (TT)
FAX (604) 431-2199

MANITOBA
1080 Portage Avenue
Winnipeg, Manitoba R3G 3M3
(800) 552-4893   (204) 774-5421
(204) 775-9802 (TT)   FAX (204) 775-5090

NEW BRUNSWICK
231 Saunders Street
Fredericton, New Brunswick E3B 1N6
(800) 270-2642   (506) 458-0060

NEWFOUNDLAND AND LABRADOR
70 The Boulevarde
St. John's, Newfoundland A1A 1K2
(709) 754-1180   FAX (708) 754-2018

NOVA SCOTIA - PRINCE EDWARD ISLAND
6136 Almon Street
Halifax, Nova Scotia B3K 1T8
(800) 565-5147   (902) 453-1480
FAX (902) 454-6570

ONTARIO
1929 Bayview Avenue
Toronto, Ontario M4G 3E8
(416) 486-2500   FAX (416) 480-7503

QUEBEC
3622 rue Ochelaga
Montreal, Quebec H1W 1J1
(800) 465-4622   (514) 529-2040
FAX (514) 529-4662

SASKATCHEWAN
2550 Broad Street
Regina, Saskatchewan S4P 3Z4
(306) 525-2571   FAX (306) 565-3300

INDEX OF ORGANIZATIONS

This index contains only those organizations listed under sections titled "ORGANIZATIONS." These organizations may also be listed as vendors of publications, tapes, and other products.

Living with Low Vision
A Resource Guide for People with Sight Loss

The only LARGE PRINT (**18 point bold type**) comprehensive guide to services and products that help individuals with vision loss throughout North America. An extremely valuable self-help tool, this guide provides people with sight loss the information they need to keep reading, working, and enjoying life. Chapters on self-help groups, making everyday living easier, and special information for children, elders, and people with vision loss and hearing loss. Information on laws that affect people with vision loss, including the ADA, and high tech equipment that promotes independence and employment. This new edition includes information about computer bulletin boards and special resources on the Internet.

Fourth edition. 1996 ISBN 0-929718-14-3 $43.95

Rehabilitation Resource Manual: VISION

A desk reference that enables professionals to make effective referrals. Includes information on the responses to vision loss; breaking the news of irreversible vision loss; guidelines on starting self-help groups; information on professional research and service organizations; plus chapters on optical and nonoptical aids; for special populations; and by eye condition/disease.

Fourth edition. 1993 ISBN 0-929718-10-0 $39.95

Providing Services for People with Vision Loss
A Multidisciplinary Perspective
Susan L. Greenblatt, Editor

Written by ophthalmologists, rehabilitation professionals, a physician who has experienced vision loss, and a sociologist, this book discusses how various professionals can work together to provide coordinated care for people with vision loss. Chapters include Vision Loss: A Patient's Perspective; Vision Loss: An Ophthalmologist's Perspective; Operating a Low Vision Aids Service; The Need for Coordinated Care; Making Referrals for Rehabilitation Services; Mental Health Services: The Missing Link; Self-Help Groups for People with Sight Loss; Aids and Techniques that Help People with Vision Loss; plus a Glossary. Also available on cassette.

1989 ISBN 0-929718-02-X $19.95

Meeting the Needs of People with Vision Loss
A Multidisciplinary Perspective
Susan L. Greenblatt, Editor

Written by rehabilitation professionals, physicians, and a sociologist, this book discusses how to provide appropriate information and how to serve special populations. Chapters include What People with Vision Loss Need to Know; Information and Referral Services for People with Vision Loss; The Role of the Family in the Adjustment to Blindness or Visual Impairment; Diabetes and Vision Loss - Special Considerations; Special Needs of Children and Adolescents; Older Adults with Vision and Hearing Losses; Providing Services to Visually Impaired Elders in Long Term Care Facilities; plus a series of Multidisciplinary Case Studies. Also available on cassette.

1991 ISBN 0-929718-07-0   **$24.95**

LARGE PRINT PUBLICATIONS

Designed for distribution by professionals to people with disabilities and chronic conditions, these publications include information on each condition, rehabilitation services, professional service providers, products, and resources that help people with disabilities and chronic conditions to live independently. Titles include "Living with Low Vision," "How to Keep Reading with Vision Loss," "Living with Age-Related Macular Degeneration," "Living with Hearing Loss," "Living with Arthritis," "After a Stroke," and "Living with Diabetic Retinopathy." Printed in 18 point bold type on ivory paper with black ink for maximum contrast. 8 1/2" by 11" Sold in minimum quantities of 25 copies per title. See order form on last page of this book for complete list of titles and prices.

Resources for Elders with Disabilities

This unique LARGE PRINT resource directory provides information about the services and products that elders with disabilities need to function independently. Printed in 18 point bold type, this book includes information on the diseases that cause common disabilities; the major rehabilitation networks; self-help groups; and legislation that affects people with disabilities. Chapters on hearing loss, vision loss, diabetes, arthritis, osteoporosis, Parkinson's disease, falls, stroke, and older workers describe assistive devices, organizations, and publications.

Second edition 1993 ISBN 0-929718-11-9   **$43.95**

A Woman's Guide to Coping with Disability

This **unique** book addresses the special needs of women with disabilities and chronic conditions, such as social relationships, sexual functioning, pregnancy, childrearing, caregiving, and employment. Special attention is paid to ways in which women can advocate for their rights with the health care and rehabilitation systems. Written for women in all age categories, the book has chapters on the disabilities that are most prevalent in women or likely to affect the roles and physical functions unique to women. Included are arthritis, diabetes, epilepsy, lupus, multiple sclerosis, osteoporosis, and spinal cord injury. Each chapter also includes information about the condition, service providers, and psychological aspects plus descriptions of organizations, publications and tapes, and special assistive devices. 1994 ISBN 0-929718-15-1 $39.95

Meeting the Needs of Employees with Disabilities

A comprehensive resource guide that provides information to help people with disabilities retain or obtain employment. Includes information on government programs and laws such as the Americans with Disabilities Act. Chapters on hearing and speech impairments, mobility impairments, visual impairment and blindness describe organizations, environmental adaptations, adaptive equipment, and services plus suggestions for a safe and friendly workplace. Case vignettes describing accommodations for employees with disabilities are an added feature of this special volume. 1993 ISBN 0-929718-13-5 $42.95

Resources for People with Disabilities and Chronic Conditions

A comprehensive resource guide with chapters on spinal cord injury, low back pain, diabetes, multiple sclerosis, hearing and speech impairments, vision impairment and blindness, and epilepsy. Each chapter includes information about the disease or condition; psychological aspects of the condition; professional service providers; environmental adaptations; assistive devices; and descriptions of organizations, publications, and products. Chapters on rehabilitation services, independent living, self-help, laws that affect people with disabilities (including the ADA), and making everyday living easier. Special information for children is also included. 1993 ISBN 0-929718--12-7 $44.95

Order form on next page

RESOURCES for REHABILITATION

33 Bedford Street, Suite 19A • Lexington, MA 02173 • 617-862-6455   FAX 617-861-7517

Our Federal Employer Identification Number is 04-2975-007

NAME _____

ORGANIZATION _____

ADDRESS _____

PHONE _____

[ ] Check or signed institutional purchase order enclosed for full amount of order. Purchase or‹
accepted from government agencies, hospitals, and universities <u>only</u>.

[ ] Mastercard/VISA Card number: _____

Signature: _____   Expiration date: _____

ALL ORDERS OF $50.00 OR LESS <u>MUST</u> BE PREPAID.

TITLE	QUANTITY		PRICE	TOTAL
Living with Low Vision: A Resource Guide...	____	X	$43.95	_____
Rehabilitation Resource Manual: VISION	____	X	39.95	_____
Providing Services for People with Vision Loss	____	X	19.95	_____
Meeting the Needs of People with Vision Loss	____	X	24.95	_____
Resources for Elders with Disabilities	____	X	43.95	_____
A Woman's Guide to Coping with Disability	____	X	39.95	_____
Meeting the Needs of Employees with Disabilities	____	X	42.95	_____
Resources for People with Disabilities and Chronic Conditions	____	X	44.95	_____

<u>MINIMUM PURCHASE OF 25 COPIES PER TITLE FOR THE FOLLOWING PUBLICATIONS</u>

Call for discount on purchases of 100 or more copies of any single title.

TITLE	QUANTITY		PRICE	TOTAL
Living with Low Vision	____	X	2.00	_____
How to Keep Reading with Vision Loss	____	X	1.75	_____
Living with Diabetic Retinopathy	____	X	1.75	_____
Aging and Vision Loss	____	X	1.25	_____
Living with Age-related Macular Degeneration	____	X	1.25	_____
Aids for Everyday Living with Vision Loss	____	X	1.25	_____
High Aids for People with Vision Loss	____	X	1.75	_____
Living with Arthritis	____	X	1.50	_____
Living with Hearing Loss	____	X	1.50	_____
After a Stroke	____	X	1.50	_____
Living with Diabetes	____	X	1.50	_____
			SUB - TOTAL	_____

SHIPPING & HANDLING: $50.00 or less, add $5.00; $50.01 to 100.00, add $8.00;
add $4.00 for each additional $100.00 or fraction of $100.00. Alaska, Hawaii,
U.S. territories, and Canada, add $3.00 to shipping and handling charges.
Foreign orders must be prepaid in U.S. currency. Please write for shipping charges.

	S/H	_____
<u>Prices are subject to change.</u>	TOTAL	$_____